STEM CELLS - LABORATORY AND CLINICAL RESEARCH

STEM CELL THERAPY AND USES IN MEDICAL TREATMENT

STEM CELLS - LABORATORY AND CLINICAL RESEARCH

STEM CELLS - LABORATORY AND CLINICAL RESEARCH

STEM CELL THERAPY AND USES IN MEDICAL TREATMENT

PRASAD S. KOKA
EDITOR

Nova Science Publishers, Inc.
New York

For permission to use material from this book please contact us:
Telephone 631-231-7269; Fax 631-231-8175
Web Site: http://www.novapublishers.com

Additional color graphics may be available in the e-book version of this book.

LIBRARY OF CONGRESS CATALOGING-IN-PUBLICATION DATA
Library of Congress Cataloging-in-Publication Data

Stem cell therapy and uses in medical treatment / editor, Prasad S. Koka.
p. cm.
Includes index.
ISBN 978-1-61324-008-3 (hardcover)
1. Stem cells. 2. Stem cells--Therapeutic use. 3. Stem cells--Transplantation. I. Koka, Prasad S.
QH588.S83S74273 2011
616'.02774--dc22
2011007690

Published by Nova Science Publishers, Inc. † New York

Contents

Preface

This new book presents and discusses current research in the study of stem cell therapy. Topics discussed include stem cell-based therapies; current therapies for multiple sclerosis; stem cell transplantation modulates mRNA gene expression profile in doxorubicin-induced cardiomyopathy; human somatic cell nuclear transfer and parthenogenesis; human cord blood stem cell applications in cell therapy; cancer stem cells and neurotrophin in obstetrics and gynecology.

Chapter 1 – The objective of this literature review is to analyse the difficulties that stem cell-based therapies may face on their way from the laboratory to the human clinical trials. Method: Review of legal and ethical requirements and the most recent articles. The paper reviews ethical and legal European requirements for biomedical research involving humans and discusses conditions for justifiable clinical trials of stem cell-based therapies with and without alternative treatment options. Results: The article discusses safety as one of the obstacles to advance stem cell-based therapies from laboratories to clinics and presents the greatest technological challenges as well as the suggested potential ways to overcome them. Results that have to be shown in animals in order to justify clinical trials of stem cell-based therapies are further discussed and the greatest challenges as well as the potential ways to overcome them are presented. The article further analyses the ethical issues related to the design of clinical trials of stem cell-based therapies and ethical problems raised by randomised clinical trials when alternative treatments exist. The question of the use of placebo control groups in such trials as well as the question of who should participate in Phase I studies of such therapies are addressed. The article then discusses other obstacles to advancing stem cell-based therapies from laboratory research to patient's bedside, such as commercial and financial obstacles, as well as different legal regulations in the EU member states. Conclusion: Suggested steps to determine the conditions for proceeding with human experimentation are presented.

Chapter 2 – Main problem: Disc degeneration is characterized by dysfunctional cells and a decrease in extra-cellular components. Transplantation of stem cells and progenitor cells may provide a new approach to treat disc degeneration. In this study the authors investigate the possibility for stem cells and progenitor cells to survive and differentiate in the non-vascularized intervertebral disc.

Methods: Bone marrow was collected from Sprague-Dawley rats and mononuclear cells isolated. The cells were labeled with a fluorescence dye and transplanted into coccygeal discs in syngeneic rats. Non-injected adjacent discs served as controls. After different time-points

(0, 7, 14 or 21 days) the discs were fixed for routine histological staining or processed for cryosections where the number of fluorescein-labeled transplanted cells was counted. Expression of collagen II was assessed using immunofluorescence technique.

Results: All cell-suspension injected discs contained transplanted bone-marrow cells. There was a decrease in detected cells at 7, 14 and 21 days compared to day 0. Transplanted cells expressed collagen II after 21 days but not after 7 and 14 days.

Conclusions: The results suggest that transplanted bone marrow-derived mononuclear cells can survive and differentiate within the intervertebral disc. Further studies in models of disc degeneration are warranted to investigate the regenerative potential of the disc following cell transplantation.

Chapter 3 – During the past decade, major advances in the treatment of multiple sclerosis (MS) have been accomplished mainly due to the introduction of immunomodulatory and immunosuppressive agents, which have significantly altered the natural course of this incurable and disabling neurodegenerative disorder. Recent studies have demonstrated the importance of the early initiation of treatment for the reduction of short-term and potentially long-term neurological impairment associated with MS. However, despite early diagnosis and early initiation of therapy, patients still experience breakthrough relapses and progression of their underlying MS pathology. The imperfect effectiveness, side effects, and toxicity of these agents, emphasize the necessity for development of more effective medications with less adverse events. It is increasingly recognized that MS progression, in addition to demyelination, leads to substantial irreversible damage to, and loss of neurons, resulting in brain atrophy and cumulative disability. One of the most promising neuroprotective strategies involves the use of bone marrow (BM) derived stem cells. Both hematopoietic and non-hematopoietic (stromal) cells can, under certain circumstances, differentiate into cells of various neuronal and glial lineages. Consequently, stem cell transplantation has been increasingly considered for the therapy-resistant MS. In this review, the status of the current therapies for MS is discussed in the context of long-term remission benefits as relates to the mechanisms of immunopathology and immunoregulation. The outcome of ongoing clinical trials, as well as of studies in patients and animal models, will help to determine the role of stem-cell transplantation in the treatment of MS. Furthermore, it seems that future therapeutic strategies for MS should combine immunomodulation with neuroprotective modalities to achieve maximal clinical benefit.

Chapter 4 – The authors previously reported that epimyocardial injection of bone marrow-derived stem cells (BMCS) inhibits cardiac remodeling and prevents further functional impairment measured 28 days after cell application in doxorubicin-induced cardiomyopathic rabbit hearts. This effect could not be attributed to transdifferentiation of donor cells. They therefore speculated that paracrine actions exerted by the BMCS might play an important role in cardiac repair and functional improvement.

When transplanted locally into doxorubicin-induced cardiomyopathic rabbits, BMCS attenuate ventricular function relative to controls. The trigger of mRNA expression may be the first response to cell transplantation. However, little is known to date about the impact of these cells on regulation of cardiomyocyte mRNA expression. In the current study the authors demonstrate that locally transplanted BMCS inhibit the doxorubicin-induced altered mRNA profiles and trigger reverse myocardial remodeling. Support for our hypothesis of a BMCS paracrine action is provided by globally enhanced mRNA expression of cardioprotective and pro-angiogenetic factors VEGF, bFGF and IGF.

In addition, the authors observed normalization of ANP mRNA levels as an indicator of improved heart function. The current study may be the first evidence that autologous BMCS may regulate gene expression profile.

Chapter 5 – The aim of the present study was to conduct preliminary experiments towards generation of autologous human embryonic stem cell lines by somatic cell nuclear transfer (SCNT) and parthenogenesis. A total of fifteen MII human oocytes were obtained from six female donors from a collaborating IVF clinic. Each woman having produced more than 20 eggs, donated 2- 3 eggs for research with written informed consent. Nine oocytes were used for SCNT and six for parthenogenesis.

For SCNT, the meiotic spindle of MII human oocytes was removed after visualization using a POLSCOPE, and the somatic cell was injected into the enucleated cytoplast, circumventing the need for electrofusion of the somatic cell and cytoplast. Six out of nine oocytes survived reconstruction during SCNT and four divided. Nuclear assessment of SCNT embryos by Hoechst 33342 staining confirmed nuclear division in some embryos post SCNT.

Parthenogenetic activation was carried out by calcium ionomycin followed by 6- DMAP treatment. All the activated eggs showed presence of pronuclei after 16 hours, four out of six oocytes showed cleavage and one embryo developed into a compacted morula. It was placed on a feeder layer but neither attached nor showed any further growth.

The authors believe the generation of autologous ES cell lines is essential to circumvent immune rejection if embryonic stem cells are to be used widely for therapy, however extensive standardization and optimization of technology is warranted.

Chapter 6 – Human umbilical cord blood (UCB) is a valuable alternative source of ethically acceptable, clinically competent stem cells that is most likely closest to embryonic stem cells. Development of reliable methods for the expansion of cord blood stem cells is critical to ensure their clinical application. In the present article, advances in cord blood stem cell isolation, culture expansion methods through co-culture with human mesenchymal stem cells, culture optimization techniques with defined media and cord blood stem cell banking aspects have been reviewed. Refined methods of isolation as well as defined culture conditions of expansion that favor retention of stem cell phenotype and proper cryogenic storage can significantly increase the use of cord blood stem cells in human cell therapy applications.

Chapter 7 – Several studies have shown the existence of cancer stem cells and suggested that they might have a role to play in chemotherapy resistance and radioresistance. Their survival skills may be the contributing factor to incomplete remission of tumors and relapse of tumors periodically followed with metastasis. The irrefutable proof of existence of cancer stem cells in hematopoietic system made way for studies with solid tumors in quest for a similar phenomenon which may be exploited to tumor therapy. Advances have been made in this field and one is poised to utilize properties of the cancer stem cells to generate fresh drugs. Recent finding suggesting ROS related genes as one of the mechanisms by which the cancer stem cells can generate resistance is a hope towards new therapeutic avenues.

Chapter 8 – complication contributing to early mortality in HIV/AIDS patients. The proto-oncogene c-mpl, identified as the thrombopoietin receptor is involved in multilineage differentiation of CD34+ hematopoietic progenitor cells. The authors have introduced the c-mpl gene into CD34+ cells via transduction of the lentivirus p156RRLsinPPTmPGK-CMPL-PRE. The lentiviral construct expresses c-mpl on approximately 90% of purified CD34+ cells. These transduced cells have then been reconstituted into human fetal thymus/liver implants in severe combined immunodeficient mice (SCID-hu Thy/Liv). The c-mpl expression on transduced CD34+ cells is not susceptible to downregulation due to the effects of HIV-1 infection. Reconstituted CD34+ cells transduced with control lentivirus, p156RRLsinPPTmPGK-EGFP-PRE, express EGFP at >90%. Reconstituted c-mpl expressing SCID-hu implants show almost maximum rescue (~90%) of myelopoiesis, erythropoiesis and megakaryopoiesis, during HIV-1 infection in vivo, at 6 weeks post-infection. The authors also show that the differentiated multi-lineage progeny colonies and thymocytes in mice reconstituted with the c-mpl transduced CD34+ cells, carry the HLA Class I loci phenotypes of these donor cells, in the implants of the recipient SCID-hu animals. The authors propose a gene therapeutic strategy, with c-mpl as the major genetic component, to address the morbidity and mortality resulting from cytopenias in HIV infected patients.

Chapter 9 – Since Rita Levi Montalcini and Stanley Cohen received Nobel Prize for their pioneering work on nerve growth factor (NGF), its role in female reproductive system has been reinforced in last two decades. The neurotrophins (NT) including nerve growth factor (NGF) are a family of related growth factors and their respective receptor tyrosine kinases that are of major importance in the regulation of neuronal survival and differentiation. While role of NGF in mast cell-mediated egg implantation and inhibition of rejection were primary concern at their time, in the ovary NGF can help in the differentiation process by which ovarian follicles become responsive to gonadotrophins. They help in follicular maturation, steroid secretion and ovulation in the ovary, by inducing the FSH receptor (FSHR). Due to the pleiotropism, NGF is mandatory for the success of pregnancy, while progesterone helping to maintain local levels of NGF in utero. In endometriosisi and polycystic ovarian disease it has major role to play. An autocrine role of NGF in breast cancer and epithelial ovarian cancer (EOC) is evident now. Thus its study will infuse new insight in diseases of both obstetrics and gynaecology.

Versions of these chapters were also published in *Journal of Stem Cells,* Volume 2, Numbers 1, 3 and 4, and Volume 2, Numbers 2, 3, and 4, edited by Prasad S. Koka, published by Nova Science Publishers, Inc. They were submitted for appropriate modifications in an effort to encourage wider dissemination of research.

In: Stem Cell Therapy and Uses in Medical Treatment
Editor: Prasad S. Koka, pp. 1-22
ISBN: 978-1-61324-008-3

Chapter 1

Stem Cell-Based Therapies: The Roadmap to the Clinic

Kristina Hug*

Department of Medical Ethics, Lund University, Sweden
Department of Health Management, Faculty of Public Health, Kaunas University of Medicine, Lithuania

Abstract

The *objective* of this literature review is to analyse the difficulties that stem cell-based therapies may face on their way from the laboratory to the human clinical trials. *Method:* Review of legal and ethical requirements and the most recent articles. The paper reviews ethical and legal European requirements for biomedical research involving humans and discusses conditions for justifiable clinical trials of stem cell-based therapies with and without alternative treatment options. *Results:* The article discusses safety as one of the obstacles to advance stem cell-based therapies from laboratories to clinics and presents the greatest technological challenges as well as the suggested potential ways to overcome them. Results that have to be shown in animals in order to justify clinical trials of stem cell-based therapies are further discussed and the greatest challenges as well as the potential ways to overcome them are presented. The article further analyses the ethical issues related to the design of clinical trials of stem cell-based therapies and ethical problems raised by randomised clinical trials when alternative treatments exist. The question of the use of placebo control groups in such trials as well as the question of who should participate in Phase I studies of such therapies are addressed. The article then discusses other obstacles to advancing stem cell-based therapies from laboratory research to patient's bedside, such as commercial and financial obstacles, as well as different legal regulations in the EU member states. *Conclusion:* Suggested steps to determine the conditions for proceeding with human experimentation are presented.

* Corresponding author: Kristina Hug. Department of Medical Ethics, BMC C 13, 221 84 Lund, Sweden. E-mail: Kristina.Hug@med.lu.se

Keywords: Human stem cells, human stem cell-based therapies, clinical trials, biomedical research ethics.

1. Introduction

Stem cells are being investigated for a long list of diseases, including Parkinson's Disease, Multiple Sclerosis, Huntington's Disease, Alzheimer's Disease, cancer of the central nervous system, spinal cord injury, retinal degenerative disorders, stroke, diabetes and trauma [1]. Like every new area of biomedical science, stem cell research is under considerable pressure from patient groups to develop human therapies as rapidly as possible. At the same time there are moral obligations to refrain from moving to first human trials until the risks involved are properly characterized in laboratory and animal studies. In stem cell research, this tension is particularly acute [2]. Four ways have been reported in which stem cell research poses unique problems when compared with other new therapeutic strategies:

1) Controversies about the use of early human embryos in research have made it politically difficult in some countries to fund research that establishes new embryonic stem cell lines. Therefore, the selection of stem cell sources for preclinical and clinical testing becomes limited by policies protecting human embryos from destruction [2].
2) Safety information about stem cells is very incomplete, partly because human stem cells have only been developed in the laboratory since 1998. Although research on human stem cells is based on 20 years of animal stem cell experiments, few safety questions relating to human applications have been addressed in animal research [2].
3) Regulatory structure and preclinical and clinical research methods used to evaluate new medical treatments are most sophisticated in the area of drug development. New and complex biological agents, like cell-based therapies, pose especially difficult problems in risk evaluation, selection of appropriate assays for clinical outcomes, and selection of study populations for early phase trials [2].
4) Hopes, expectations, and misconceptions may influence the objectivity of both the research participant's and the research investigator's decision-making ability. It is a challenge to create processes to ensure the safety of patients and research participants due to the following pressures [3]:

(a) *The division of opinions regarding the use of human embryonic and foetal tissue to develop stem cell lines for research.* In a number of countries the destruction of a human embryo in order to isolate embryonic stem cells is seen as a wrongdoing. This issue, however, has already been discussed in the previous articles of the author.

(b) *The "overselling" of outcomes as a result of the researcher's desire to be the first to discover a cellular therapy.* Researcher's too optimistic hope for the outcome of the study may result in "overselling" of the potential benefits of the study. The researcher may feel the pressure to benefit of publishing papers and assure tenure at a university setting [3].

(c) *Therapeutic misconception resulting from a clinical trial participant's desire for a miracle cure.* Unrealistic hopes have resulted from great enthusiasm for these discoveries before scientific bases and proofs are available. Research participants often suffer from a "therapeutic misconception" that there is a possibility of receiving a therapeutic benefit by participating in research. As the physician assumes a different role as principal investigator, the existing doctor-patient relationship of trust may result in the patients reviewing the consent documents with less depth, under the assumption that it must be good for them if recommended by their trusted physician. In addition, the physician's enthusiasm for the trial as a researcher may result in a patient participating in a study out of loyalty to the physician and/or therapeutic misconception [3].

The above-mentioned problems need to be discussed and given a reasonable solution before human clinical trials of stem cell-based treatments are stared. The arguments for and against the need to establish new stem embryonic cell lines as well as the attitudes to stem cell research in different countries will be discussed in another article. This article will analyse the following issues:

1) The conditions under which clinical trials of stem cell-based therapies with and without alternative treatment options can be justified;
2) The results that have to be shown in animals in order to justify clinical trials of such therapies;
3) The design of the clinical trials of stem cell-based therapies and the ethical problems raised by randomised clinical trials when alternative treatments exist;
4) Obstacles that make it difficult to advance stem cell-based therapies from laboratory research to patient's bedside.

2. The Conditions under Which Clinical Trials of Stem Cell-Based Therapies with and without Alternative Treatment Options Can Be Justified

It has been reported that there are signs that stem cells could emerge as an important issue to the industry: at least eight different treatments involving adult stem cells are already in use, and more than a dozen adult cell, umbilical cord and foetal cell therapies are in clinical trials. Furthest along in commercial development are adult cells [4]. For example, *Nature Biotechnology* magazine lists 37 companies worldwide working on foetal or adult stem cells. Virtually all are small biotechnology companies, with about half of them in human trials or on the market already, and the rest of them at earlier stages of studying in the laboratories or in animals [4]. Regarding human trials of stem cell-based treatments, concern has been expressed that researchers may place sick patients at risk if clinical trials are started too early. For example, it has been argued that scientists still do not know exactly:

- Which kinds of stem cells work best in treating certain pathology;
- How and when it is best to implant them;
- What the cells do once they are implanted;

- What kinds of patients are the best candidates for early stage clinical trials [5].

What are the legal and ethical requirements for the justifiable start of clinical trials on humans? Table 1 provides a brief overview what the main European documents say regarding the justification of clinical trials.

Are human clinical trials of stem cell-based therapies ready to fulfil these requirements? The following main concerns can be expressed:

- Regarding Art. 11 of the Helsinki Declaration – can the scientists honestly state that thorough knowledge based on adequate laboratory and animal experimentation already exists? Chapter 4 of this article will discuss what is still left to be proved by animal experimentation in order to justify clinical trials of stem cell-based therapies.

Table 1. Ethical and legal European requirements for biomedical research involving human subjects

Document	Biomedical research involving human subjects can be ethically justifiable only if:
Art. 5, Helsinki Declaration [6]	The well-being of the human subject takes precedence over the interests of science and society [6].
Art. 6, Helsinki Declaration [6]	The primary purpose is to improve prophylactic, diagnostic and therapeutic procedures and the understanding of disease aetiology and pathogenesis [6].
Art. 11, Helsinki Declaration [6]	Research conforms to generally accepted scientific principles, is based on a thorough knowledge of the scientific literature and on adequate laboratory and animal experimentation [6].
Art. 17, Helsinki Declaration [6]	Physicians are confident that the risks involved have been adequately assessed and can be satisfactorily managed. Physicians should cease any investigation if the risks are found to outweigh the potential benefits or if there is conclusive proof of positive and beneficial results [6].
Art. 18, Helsinki Declaration [6] Art. 3 (2a), Clinical Trials Directive [2] Art 15 (7), Advanced Therapy Directive [8] Guideline 8, CIOMS Guidelines [9]	The importance of the objective outweighs the inherent risks and burdens *to the subject* [6]. The foreseeable risks and inconveniences have been weighed against the anticipated benefit for the individual *trial subject and other present and future patients* [7]. Risk management system designed to identify, prevent or minimise risks related to advanced therapy medicinal products, including an evaluation of the effectiveness of that system, is set up (where there is cause for concern) [8]. Potential benefits and risks are reasonably balanced and risks are minimized. Interventions or procedures that hold out the prospect of direct therapeutic benefit for the individual subject must be justified by the expectation that they will be *at least as advantageous to the individual subject as any available alternative.* Risks of such "beneficial" interventions or procedures must be justified in relation to expected benefits to the individual subject [9].
Art. 9 (5), Clinical Trials Directive [7]	Written authorisation is given before the commencement of clinical trials on medicinal products the active ingredient(s) of which is or are a biological product or biological products of human or animal origin, or contains biological components of human or animal origin, or the manufacturing of which requires such components [7].
Art. 5 (1), Cells and Tissue Directive [10] Commentary to CIOMS Guideline 1 [9]	Tissue and cell procurement and testing are carried out by persons with appropriate training and experience and take place in conditions accredited, designated, authorised or licensed for that purpose by the competent authority/authorities [10]. All who participate in the conduct of research are qualified by virtue of their education and experience to perform competently in their roles [9].
Guideline 1, CIOMS Guidelines [9]	It is carried out in ways that respect and protect, and are fair to, the subjects of that research and are morally acceptable within the communities in which the research is carried out [9].

- Regarding Art. 17 of the Helsinki Declaration – do the scientists agree that the risks involved in such clinical trials have been adequately assessed and can be satisfactorily managed? Chapter 3 of this article will discuss the obstacles that make it difficult to transfer stem cell-based therapies from laboratory to patient's bedside. The issue of safety is an especially important one.
- Even if many scientists agree that the importance of the objective of this kind of research outweighs the inherent risks and burdens to the subject, as required by Art. 18 of the Helsinki Declaration, does the scientific community today agree that interventions with the prospect of direct therapeutic benefit for the individual subject are justified by the expectation that they will be at least as advantageous to the individual subject as any available alternative? This concern is, of course, relevant to cases where alternative treatment options do exist. What kind of trial design should be applied in such clinical trials? Chapter 5 of this article will discuss this issue in greater detail.
- Regarding CIOMS Guideline 1 – will clinical trials of embryonic stem cell-based therapies be morally acceptable within the communities in which these trials are carried out? This particular question has already been analysed by previous articles of the author and therefore will not be discussed in detail here. Chapter 6 of this article, however, presents the problems related to different legal regulations in the European Community.

3. Safety as an Obstacle to Advance Stem Cell-Based Therapies from Laboratories to Patient's Bedside

Before clinical trials of human stem cells (especially embryonic ones, the research on which is the least advanced) for therapeutic applications are thinkable, several issues have to be resolved. First of all, the use of stem cells must be safe [11]. Care must be taken in translating lab-based experimental results into the clinic because premature human trials could be damaging to both the patients and the field of cell-based therapies in general [12].

Amongst the greatest technological challenges there are the following issues:

1) *Immunocompatibility.* Transplanted cells could be subject to immune system rejection and in some cases may cause graft versus host disease [2]. Even if the transplantation of embryonic stem cells is already performed on mouse models, these biotechnologies cannot yet be applied to humans before it is shown that the transfer of an alien gene will not cause immunological reaction and thus the rejection of the alien protein [13]. Further research is required to characterize the cellular and humeral immune response to engrafted human embryonic stem cells [14].

This challenge can potentially be overcome by a variety of strategies (besides treating the graft recipient with immunosuppressive drugs, which can be associated with unpleasant side effects and render the patient susceptible to infection) [2, 11]:

(a) *Using patient's own cells* (e.g. adult stem cells taken from the patient's bone marrow) [4].
(b) *Establishing large banks of embryonic stem cells that would enable selection of cells* which would result in the possibility to find a best immunological fit for the patient in question [13, 14, 15]. It has been argued, however, that the creation of such a stem cell bank is probably not feasible [11]. Some authors have suggested that more than 1 million cell lines might be required for ensuring chances of finding a matching cell line for a patient [16]. Embryonic stem cell grafts from such cell lines would likely still encounter rejection, as research on mice shows [17].
(c) *Making embryonic stem cells to an individual patient by:*

- Somatic cell nuclear transfer (therapeutic cloning), where human embryonic stem cells are derived from an embryo that was cloned from the patient's own tissues and are then used for autologous transplantation [15, 18]. Such stem cells would be perfectly compatible to the treated patient, as they would carry the patient's genome [19, 20]. This solution, however, gives rise to problems from both the technical and the ethical point of view [13].
- Sophisticated methods for "transplanting" human leukocyte antigen (HLA) regions from the patient's genome to embryonic stem cells [21].

(d) Generating "universal" embryonic stem cell lines by removing genetic components that trigger the immune system of most human recipients [13, 15, 21]. Genetic modification of embryonic stem cells provides a means to reduce their immunological incompatibility. This could be achieved by inserting immune-osuppressive molecules or by deleting immunoreactive molecules [22]. A resulting cell line would then not induce rejection or will induce just minor immune responses. However, the creation of such a "universal" stem cell remains technically out of reach at present and in the foreseeable future [2, 14].
(e) Replacing foreign major histocompatability complex genes by the recipient's corresponding genes, increasing the immunological compatibility of the cells [22].
(f) Using the same human embryonic stem cell line to derive both lympho-haematopoietic stem cells and the therapeutic cell type required for transplantation, and transplantation of the lympho-haematopoietic stem cells is carried out first so that immune tolerance would be achieved before the second transplant [15].
(g) Modulating the recipient's immune system in a way that the desired cells are not being rejected [23, 24, 25] by inducing specific lifelong transplantation tolerance. There are indications in humans that this approach may be effective [14].
(h) Conducting animal studies to clarify whether there are immunologic reactions to foreign tissue in the central nervous system [2]. It is established that the brain is immunologically privileged (immune activity in the brain is suppressed) as compared with other sites [26]. For example, some investigators have described unique and specialized immune system regulation within the central nervous system [27], where immune activation markers may be expressed at low levels [2]. Therefore it is not clear whether immunosuppression is needed in allograft situations.

2) *Misdifferentiation.* Cells may differentiate *in vivo* into undesirable cell types or fail to express the properties of the fully differentiated cells that are needed for therapeutic purposes [2]. The effects of misdifferentiation are extremely difficult to predict and pose both short-term and long-term largely unknown risks to potential human subjects [2]. For example, it is not known whether cells can "de-differentiate" after selection and transplantation, forming tissue types other than that which was intended [2]. The risk of implanting undifferentiated embryonic stem cells or inappropriate cell lineages can further cause tumour formation or further perturbation of tissue function [22]. Animal experiments have showed that embryonic stem cells infused in some parts of the body might start making different types of tissues, all the way to forming cancers [4].

This challenge can potentially be overcome by determining which genes are activated during various phases of differentiation and finding molecules that will help the cells stay differentiated the right way [4]. If this is known, then a patient could have a gene inserted that would kill the misdifferentiating cell if the patient were given a particular drug. If the stem cell began differentiating wildly or turning malignant, the patient could be given this "trigger drug" [2, 4]. Such a "suicide gene strategy" is promising in the development of human cell therapies, but more investigation is needed. An open question is whether first human trials should wait until this "suicide gene strategy" is available [2]. From the ethical point of view, it is also unclear whether it is acceptable to transplant patients with cells which have been genetically modified with a suicide gene.

3) *Mistargeting.* Even when cells differentiate properly, there is no guarantee that they will not miss the target and will not migrate to other tissues or organs, potentially causing dangerous side effects [2].
   This challenge can potentially be overcome by more animal testing for gaining better understanding of the processes of differentiation and migration [2].
4) *Tumour formation.* Transplanted cells have the potential to form tumours as a result of inadequate regulation of cell division [2]. For example, human embryonic stem cells, when transplanted directly into the brain, can form solid tumours [28].

This challenge can potentially be overcome by:

- *Manipulating embryonic stem cells first in vitro* to direct them to differentiate in a desired way [12]. It may be that risks of tumour formation are greater in cases where the transplanted cells are not fully differentiated. Yet for some therapeutic applications, it may be preferable to have final maturation of cells occur *in vivo*, rather than in laboratory culture [2].
- *In some cases, using immunosuppression in patients* would allow more rapid formation and detection of tumours [2].
- *Making predictions about tumour-formation qualities of individual cell lines* based on their degree of differentiation and homogeneity with respect to specific markers [2].
- *Transplanting only differentiated cells* to avoid the risk of cancer formation in the recipient [23].

5) *The danger of transmitting infections.* The existing human embryonic stem cell lines are not ideal for clinical use, as the majority of cell lines reported worldwide have been derived from mouse fibroblast feeder layers. Direct contact with the mouse feeders makes these lines as xenotransplantation products [14] and any potential therapy developed from these lines carries the possibility of cross-species transfer of infections [29]. In addition, the screening of embryo donors in the past was not always strictly performed, and the cells may also have been exposed to materials derived from animal species [14]. It has been argued, however, that stem cells do not pose any greater risk of infection than any other tissue or organ transplant [29].

This challenge can potentially be overcome by:

- *Screening to protect recipients from infectious agents* (either human adventitious agents or animal-derived pathogens) [29]. Rules for xenotransplantation should be applied, which would include specific testing and sampling requirements to assess the risks of infectious disease, as well as specific requirements to inform potential research subjects about these risks and about the need to abstain from blood or tissue donation after receiving a xenotransplant [30].
- *Creating reliable ways to grow human stem cell lines without mouse feeder layers* [31, 32]. It would mean that it would be necessary to derive new human embryonic stem cell lines using a non-animal culture system [14]. It has been demonstrated that the use of mouse feeders may be replaced by propagation of human embryonic stem cells on extra-cellular matrices in the presence of a mouse embryonic, fibroblast-conditioned medium [33]. Although this system avoids direct contact between mouse feeders and human embryonic stem cells, the risk of cross-transfer of animal pathogens from the animal-conditioned medium to the human embryonic stem cells is not avoided [33]. An alternative could be to use human feeders, combined with animal-free reagents to support the derivation and propagation of human embryonic stem cell lines [34, 35].
- *Establishing good manufacturing practices and quality control procedures* for stem cell lines that will potentially be used for future cell therapies [2]. Appropriate standards and assays will need to be developed to test stability of the potentially immortal stem cell lines that can continuously be used in the laboratory for many generations. Good manufacturing procedures must be established for every step of the development of specific derivatives of these cell lines to be used in human trials [2].

6) *The danger of transmitting genetic disorders.* This risk is difficult to evaluate. In the absence of animal and human trials, it is not clear how specific cells will behave after transplant [2].

This challenge can potentially be overcome by:

- *Screening donor tissue for genetic disorders that would be directly relevant to the proposed use of the stem cells,* such as type I diabetes for islet transplant [2]. It remains to be determined how much genetic screening should be done on a routine basis or whether donor tissue should be excluded if a genetic mutation unrelated to the disease being treated is present. A key question is what, if any, genetic mutations stem cell lines should be tested for, in addition to those believed to be directly relevant to the intended therapeutic function of the cells [2].

- *Collecting family medical histories from couples who are willing to donate leftover embryos* in infertility clinics [2]. It can be argued, however, that such a practice would burden potential donors with additional tasks, which could negatively affect their wish to donate.

Bearing in mind the risks mentioned above, the following issues still remain unsolved:

1) *There is considerable uncertainty about both the magnitude and probability of the risks that the first human subjects will face* even if only new, quality controlled stem cell lines are used, and even if first human trials follow extensive preclinical testing [2].
2) *It is not clear how to measure the safety and toxicity of stem cell grafts in human beings.* The kinds of assays used in testing new pharmacologic agents, such as drug metabolites, blood chemistry, and liver enzyme levels, may not be entirely relevant [2].
3) *It may be difficult to assess location and function on a cellular level,* since many of the histological tests used in preclinical testing would largely be impossible in human patients, except in autopsy cases [2]. This challenge could possibly be overcome by using imaging techniques that may be available to observe changes in metabolic activity in specific tissue areas. But even using this technology it is impossible to determine which cells caused these metabolic changes or what their specific phenotypes and functions are [2].
4) *It is questionable whether longer follow-up periods and patient registries should be established for stem cell trials* [2]. It has been argued that model protocols designed to capture long-term risks should be designed, paying much attention to collecting sufficient follow-up data relating to adverse events [2].

It has been predicted that due to the number and severity of the technological challenges remaining to be solved before the initiation of large scale clinical trials, human embryonic stem cells are not likely to be a part of routine clinical practise in the near future [23].

4. Results That Have to Be Shown in Animals in Order to Justify Clinical Trials of Stem Cell-Based Therapies

The question of how much animal testing should be required before human trials may ethically proceed is difficult to resolve, given that cell-based therapy is a relatively new one and appropriate assays and outcomes have yet to be defined [2]. There is currently a lack of data from animal experiments regarding certain risks, and, in some cases, a lack of good animal models for testing, as some risks can only be fully assessed using *in vivo* testing. It has been reported that *at least four types of risks will need to be evaluated with preclinical animal testing,* and in the future, in early phase human trials [2]:

1. The risk of “misdifferentiation”;
2. The risk of “mistargeting”;
3. The risk of tumour formation;
4. Immune system rejection [2].

It has been argued that the decisions on what types of animal experiments are required before clinical trials are likely to be made on a case-to-case basis [23]. The complexity of the required animal studies depends on the type of patients being tested as well as the ability to remove the transplanted cells if unwanted side effects should appear [23].

Amongst the greatest challenges there are the following issues:

1) The use of animal stem cells in animal experiments will not necessarily answer questions about specific human stem cell lines or their derivatives. Given that successful methods of culturing and differentiating cells vary from one species to the next, the extent to which it is reasonable to extrapolate from test results with mouse cell lines to human cell lines is unclear [2]. For example, although mouse models of human disease have proven extremely valuable in understanding many diseases, a critical problem is whether mouse or rat models truly mimic human injury in their etiology and progression [36]. It has been argued that since animal models are not likely to provide clear-cut answers, we should go ahead and transplant in humans already now [36]. Patient advocates have argued strongly that in diseases where death is inevitable and where volunteers exist perhaps we should do this. At the very worst we will have learned something that will be useful and perhaps we will have a spectacular success [36]. However, it has also been suggested that the available results argue against a spectacular success and the lack of caution may do more harm than good [36]. Unless animal model systems are developed that highly resemble the planned clinical trial, animal studies will only be of limited value to predict toxic side effects of using human stem cells or their derivatives [23].
2) Determining what methods to use to monitor cell fate and performance as well as post-implantation outcomes. The parameters that would need to be assessed are cell migration and differentiation, cell phenotypes expressed, functional integration of cells, and post-implantation cell survival [2]. There are as yet no standard assays for these outcomes [2]. However, various imaging techniques such as MRI will be valuable for following the fate, including migration, differentiation and function, of the transplanted cells in the living patient.
3) The potential for tumour formation is difficult to characterize in animal experiments. It has been argued that in some cases tumour formation may only occur over long periods, and small animals have short life spans [2]. Experiments involving larger species are expensive and, for some, more ethically problematic. Moreover, it could take decades to establish with confidence the risk of tumour genesis in, for example,

nonhuman primates [2]. Nevertheless, follow-up times in animal experiments have to take into account the problem of potential tumour formation [2].

Various imaging techniques such as MRI will be valuable for following the fate, including migration, differentiation and function, of the transplanted cells in the living patient. This should be pointed out in the text.

These challenges can potentially be overcome by:

1) *Both same-species and inter-species testing* to determine the relevance of species-specific signalling and host environment and to select the most appropriate animal models for human disease [2].
2) *Testing human cell-based therapies in at least two different animal models before testing in human trials.* It has been argued that although this is appropriate for determining the behaviour of specific human cell lines before human use, it may be problematic to interpret the data from these experiments, given that cell-cell signalling, targeting, and response to other biochemical signals may all depend on species-specific signals [2].
3) *Considering primate models to predict human cell behaviour based on animal transplant models prior to initiating transplant studies in humans.* It has been estimated that primate models are likely to be better as their physiological parameters and many of the fundamental properties of cells are similar, and the likelihood of similar results being obtained in human studies will be higher than when extrapolating from rodent studies [36]. However, it should not be expected that dependence solely on primate studies can hasten the advent to the clinic. The advantages that make rodents so useful (e.g., the ability to make transgenic animals, the relatively low costs compared to primates, the short life span, and the numbers available for studies) and the lack of evidence that species differences will not constitute an equally intractable issue when studies are performed in primates, argue against this approach as a simple solution [36]. Primate models will be critical as a component of a staged careful approach to transplant therapy but cannot resolve all problems [36].
4) *Building on what we know to understand what we do not know and taking a step-by-step approach.* For example, treating Parkinson's disease by cell therapy can be evaluated in terms of:

   (a) which cells researchers should use,
   (b) how researchers should scale up for therapy
   (c) when the cells should be transplanted,
   (d) how far the cells will migrate,
   (e) what the caveats of the animal model are,
   (f) how researchers can test the immune issues, and so on [36].

Each component/question can be tested rigorously and in isolation to build up a predictive picture of the use of cells for treatment of Parkinson's disease [36]. At each stage a specific animal model is likely to be appropriate [36]. For example, to rule out intrinsic physiological variables, perhaps side-by-side transplants of human and rodent cells into the same model will have to be performed. It has been suggested that to study the immune response, immune-suppressed, and non-suppressed animals will have to be compared, and to study surgical techniques, diffusion, and growth rates of cells, primate models may be most appropriate [36]. Because many of these issues do not require long-term studies these can be accomplished in short order and optimized strategies can then be utilized in long-term studies. This approach is more likely to lead to clinical intervention more rapidly [36].

5) *Multiple testing and retesting and maintaining a common readily accessible database of results (including negative ones).* It is important to have careful documentation of the cells used, their physiologic state, and choice of readouts to progress from a descriptive approach to a more focused therapeutic approach [36].
6) *Testing each component of a transplant experiment separately and carefully before the entire experiment is carried out in a disease model.* For example, testing the behaviour of cells in the normal environment, testing them in multiple abnormal states, and testing worst-case scenarios (e.g., tumour formation) directly [36]. When extrapolating from one system to another, track must be kept of known anatomical, physiological, biochemical, and pharmacological differences between human and the chosen animal specie's cells [36].

In the area of stem cell research, it remains questionable how long the testing on animals should take. There are no established rules so far. Regarding the testing of drug toxicity, however, Art. 4 of the ICH Guideline on Duration of Chronic Toxicity Testing in Animals requires that the studies on rodents should last at least 6 months, and the studies on non-rodents – at least 9 months [37].

Due to the number and severity of the technological challenges remaining to be solved before the initiation of large scale clinical trials, human embryonic stem cells are not likely to be a part of routine clinical practise in the near future [23].

5. The Design of the Clinical Trials of Stem Cell-Based Therapies and the Ethical Problems Raised by Randomised Clinical Trials When Alternative Treatments Exist

Meantime many devastating diseases have been suggested as possible candidates for stem cell therapy, it has been argued that careful consideration needs to be given to the design of clinical studies [38]. So far the randomized controlled trial is the preferred methodology to identify causes, and it is called "the scientific gold standard", but from an ethical perspective it may be problematic for early-stage studies of stem cell-based therapies [38]. For example, a great deal of criticism has been expressed regarding double blind, placebo-controlled foetal neural cell transplant trials that were conducted in patients with advanced Parkinson's disease in the USA [39]. Patients in the placebo arm were subjected to sham neurosurgery which involved drilling holes into their skulls, and many bioethicists and clinicians have expressed concern about exposing patients to such risks where there is no possibility of benefit [40]. These trials have also been criticised on methodological grounds: concerns have been expressed that the inclusion of the sham surgery control group did not make the trials more scientifically valid than had they simply included a control group who had received medical treatment [38].

The use of placebo control groups in stem cell clinical trials. It has been argued that where the experimental treatment involves invasive surgery - as it will in many applications of stem cell medicine - the control treatment should not be sham surgery but the current clinically approved treatment and standard of care [38]. *Note of clarification to Art. 29 of the Helsinki Declaration*, however, states that placebo-controlled trial may be ethically acceptable even if proven therapy is available (and even in cases where risks are not minimal), if for compelling and scientifically sound methodological reasons the use of placebo is necessary to determine the efficacy or safety of a prophylactic, diagnostic or therapeutic method [6]. *Does stem cell research provide these compelling methodological reasons?*

Guideline 11 of the CIOMS Guidelines also states that although, as a general rule, research subjects in the control group of a trial of therapeutic intervention should receive an established effective intervention, placebo may still be used in the following cases:

1) When there is no established effective intervention;
2) When withholding an established effective intervention would expose subjects to temporary discomfort or delay in relief of symptoms;
3) When use of an established effective intervention as comparator would not yield scientifically reliable results and use of placebo would not add any risk of serious or irreversible harm to the subjects [9].

Considering the above-stated requirements, it can be argued that stem cell research falls only under the requirement of point 1 of the Guideline. However, would it be acceptable to use a placebo even if such use contradicts the requirements under points 2 and 3 of the Guideline? The *Commentary on CIOMS Guideline 11* further explains that a placebo-controlled design may be ethically acceptable when the condition for which research subjects are randomly assigned to placebo or active treatment is only a small deviation in physiological measurements and if delaying or omitting available treatment may cause no serious adverse consequences [9]. However, this does not seem to be the case in stem cell research. *But can there be alternative models to placebo controlled trials, models which satisfy both ethical and methodological concerns?*

Commentary on CIOMS Guideline 11 explains that placebo-control group need not be untreated and an add-on design may be employed when the investigational therapy and a standard treatment have different mechanisms of action. The treatment to be tested and placebo are each added to a standard treatment [9]. However, this approach is only possible where the standard therapy exists. In the cases of stem cell research, aimed to such clinical conditions like Alzheimer's disease, there is no standard therapy and thus an add-on design would not be possible.

The issue of using placebo, however, appears in later phases of clinical trials. The first question to be answered will be *who should participate in Phase I studies of potential stem cell-based therapies?* Before this question can be answered, it is important to recall the different characteristics of the four phases of clinical trials. Table 2 presents a brief overview of the main differences between these four phases.

When trying to answer the question who should participate in Phase I stem cell trials, another question arises: *are there some characteristics that would make it more ethically acceptable to have some people, and not others, bear the burdens of Phase I studies?* The following groups of potential participants can be considered:

Table 2. Phases of clinical trials and their features

Phase number	What is being tested	Kind of research persons
Phase I	First testing of new agents in humans, testing side effects, toxicity, and in some cases, determining the maximum tolerable dose [2].	Healthy volunteers
Phase II	Collection of further data on safety and on efficacy for the purpose of directing continuing research on the intervention, if warranted [2].	Patients
Phase III	Compares new agents to existing interventions, if any, in a larger population that is sufficient for robust statistical analysis [2].	Patients
Phase IV	Post-marketing or surveillance research conducted after regulatory approval for the purpose of obtaining safety and efficacy information from larger population groups [2].	Patients

1) *Enrolling healthy volunteers.* It has been argued that it is unlikely that Phase I stem cell trials will be conducted on healthy volunteers [2]. From a technical point of view, healthy people are not the intended target for stem cell interventions and thus they would not be sufficiently informative research subjects [2].

2) *Enrolling patients.* It has been argued that in theory, Phase I stem cell trials might offer some prospect of clinical benefit even to the first participants [2]. Therefore the model of recruiting Phase I trial human subjects from among seriously ill patients for whom medicine has nothing to offer (this model is used in oncology trials) seems appropriate. It has also been argued, however, that it is ethically unacceptable to ask patients to refuse treatments that are even partially effective in order to participate in Phase I trials, because the risks are very unclear and there is no way of assessing how likely it is that the first human experiments will work as planned [2]. Would that imply that enrolment in Phase I studies should be restricted to *patients who* do not have *meaningful alternative treatments?* Ethical documents suggest that *where no other treatment is available, high-risk experimental treatments are justified.* For example, *Art. 32 of the Helsinki Declaration* states: Where proven therapeutic methods do not exist or have been ineffective, the physician, with informed consent from the patient, must be free to use unproven or new therapeutic measures, if in the physician's judgement it offers hope of saving life, re-establishing health or alleviating suffering [6]. *Commentary to CIOMS Guideline 8* states that non-beneficial interventions may be justified only by appeal to the knowledge to be gained and it is important to consider the harm that could result from non-conducting

of the research [9]. From the above-mentioned statements it seems that the enrolment of the sickest patients who do not have any viable treatment options is a suitable answer to the question about who should be asked to participate in Phase I stem cell trials. However, is this always the case?

3) *Enrolling the sickest patients.* In early human stem cell trials, enrolling the sickest patients may not always make the best scientific sense for the following reasons:

(a) *Gravely ill patients may not be ideal for early trials for medical reasons* [2]. For example, in a controlled study of foetal cell transplants for Parkinson's disease, patients younger than 60 had a positive response to the surgery, at least at 1-year follow-up, as compared with older patients, who experienced no benefit [41].
(b) *Older or more seriously ill patients may not be the best technical choice for certain clinical trials, as longer follow-up times may be necessary* to characterize both safety and effectiveness [2]. The need to characterize long-term risks emerges in the transition from early human research to trials of later phases and to approved human therapies [2].
(c) *In some cases, proof of concept and clinical effectiveness may be difficult to establish in patients with advanced disease.* Scientific objections to enrolling the seriously ill may also provide grounds for moral concern [2].
(d) *The imperative to avoid exploitation and therapeutic misconception.* Even if researchers are scrupulous in insisting that early trials are not expected to produce any clinical benefits to participants, patients may be manipulated by their own emotions into believing that the experimental intervention can make a miracle [2]. The emotional tensions are also significant for physician-investigators who must balance honesty with compassion and with their felt duty to support an optimistic mindset among their seriously ill patients [2].
(e) *The sickest patients may often happen to be incompetent ones.* According to *Guideline 9 of the CIOMS Guidelines*, when research is conducted on individuals incapable of giving informed consent, the risk from research interventions with no prospect of direct benefit for the individual subject should be no more likely and not greater than the risk of routine medical examination of such persons. Slight or minor increases above such risk may be permitted when there is an overriding scientific or medical rationale for such increases [9]. However, the risks in Phase I stem cell clinical trials are too unclear to be categorised as "minimal", and thus it can be argued that incompetent patients may not be good candidates for Phase I clinical trials in the field of stem cell research.
(f) *Even if patients are competent, concerns about the validity of informed consent that is obtained from desperate research subjects* argue in favour of enrolling the less seriously ill in early trials, at least in some cases [2].

6. Other Obstacles to Advancing Stem Cell-Based Therapies from Laboratory Research to Patient's Bedside

The advancement of stem cell-based therapies into the clinic encounters certain *commercial and financial obstacles*. These obstacles are as follows:

1) Stem cell-based therapy, using patients' own cells rather than a patentable drug or medical device raise little commercial interest. This is especially true if the treatment can be performed with equipment already in wide use [5]. However, some device makers are helping to sponsor research on the new therapy in hopes of expanding product sales [5].
2) Financial considerations influence the development of clinical protocols, because funding is often limited. Financial incentives, personal investment in companies funding research activities, and fundraising pressures may present potential conflicts. The increasing role of emerging biotechnology and pharmaceutical companies in clinical research introduces additional financial considerations [3].
3) The shift from public to private funding of medical research adds pressures to universities and researchers seeking funds because the goals of scientific discovery are different and often conflicting in the academic and corporate settings. The research process relies on academic institutions' participation in studies leading to the development of new drugs and therapies [3]. Avoidance of the public funding process becomes even more attractive for researchers as private funding may offer researchers an opportunity to conduct research activities with less strict reporting requirements than those required with public funding [3]. Patients may also be attracted away from academic institutions and toward private trials offering greater accessibility and faster results [42]. Concerns have been expressed, however, that efficacy and safety of new treatments should be analyzed and maintained in the academic instead of private setting, as the academic setting would be more free from financial, political, and public conflicts of interest [3]. New pressures arise as activities increase in the private funding world. In the private world, the research team may face conflicting pressures, one to maintain regulatory compliance and safety, and another – to get the product to market quickly, as delays carry high costs [3]. The desire to get the results quickly may compromise research participants' safety, when decisions are made about establishing a minimum number of participants in the study, determining appropriate starting doses for the trial, and deciding the tests used to monitor efficacy of the product [3]. It has been suggested that with each of these types of decisions, safety must be balanced with the length of the study [3].
4) If reimbursement arrangements (e.g. granting patents for biotechnological inventions) are slow to follow discoveries, treatment may not be truly available to all participants of clinical trials [3]. It has been argued that legislation restricting embryonic stem cell research and limiting its funding would prolong the path to new treatments for presently incurable diseases [23]. For example, only a handful of

companies are known to be investigating embryonic stem cells [4]. It has also been argued, however, that if embryonic stem cell research receives fewer funds, other strategies for curing the same and perhaps even other diseases can receive more financial support [23]. Opinion has been expressed that these alternative strategies may perhaps reveal even better results, as it is difficult to predict the future usefulness of embryonic stem cells [23].

5) Direct relationship between the principal investigator and the funding company raises concerns of conflicting interests [3]. However, it has been difficult to agree what should be defined as a "direct relationship" and difficult to set the reasonable boundaries of restrictions. For example, questions have been raised whether a spouse of the principal investigator be restricted from financial relationships with funding entities? In a university setting, should trustees of the university disclose their financial relationships? Should all who have access to the minutes of these discussions be restricted from financial interests? Would an applicant for a training fellowship, or his or her spouse, be allowed to hold financial interest in a biotechnology company sponsoring a clinical trial [3]? It will be a challenge to develop policies to minimize financial conflicts, but operate within reason [3]. Attention has been drawn that it has also to be considered that extension of such policies may become deterrent for researchers to enter the field of research [3].

The scientific progress associated with stem cell therapy does not enter a regulatory vacuum [38] and the advancement of stem cell-based therapies in the EU also faces the obstacle created by *different legal regulations in the EU member states.* For example, if embryonic stem cells and related products are prohibited in Member State X and not prohibited in Member States Y and Z, then products based on embryonic stem cells can be developed only in Member States Y and Z, but not in X [43]. These products can be marketed only in Member States Y and Z, but not in X [43].

There are several regulatory problems that have not yet been unanimously decided by the EU member states:

(a) Regulating early clinical trials that involve unfamiliar scientific risks associated with new types of tissue transplants [38];
(b) A disunited European approach to market approval due to the uncertain borderline between a product and a device [38];
(c) Uncertainties about patentability [38];
(d) Cultural differences about the moral significance of a human embryo;
(e) Doubts about the appropriateness of holding out financial rewards or incentives for tissue donation [38];
(f) Methods of enforcement and compliance [38].

These difficulties raise the question of whether the existing regulatory framework is adequate. It has been argued that a special regulatory regime is needed for stem cell research or therapy or both in order to maintain public confidence [38]. It has also been argued that perhaps instead of yet another regulatory body all that is needed is better coordination of the existing regulations and regulators as well as more accessible descriptions of current ethical and legal standards [38]. For example, Art. 20 of the Clinical Trials Directive already foresees such an adaptation procedure: “This Directive shall be adapted to take account of scientific and technical progress” [7].

Conclusions

In the face of new and uncertain risks, especially when the clinical benefit of stem cell-based treatments has yet to be demonstrated, it is difficult to determine the conditions under which it is reasonable from an ethical point of view to proceed with human experimentation [2]. In order to determine these conditions, the following steps have been suggested:

1) *Developing specific criteria for safety and toxicity testing in Phase I stem cell clinical trials* for determining ways to measure the differentiation, migration, and function of cells after transplantation [2].
2) *Considering the following, when selecting the first human subjects for Phase I stem cell clinical trials:*

    (a) It should be avoided to enrol in first human trials patients who have clinically viable alternatives [2].
    (b) It may be considered to enrol the more seriously ill patients in cases where there is great uncertainty about risk or the biggest worry about tumour formation or other longer term consequences. However, gravely ill patients should not participate in trials if the data that are obtained are of no or limited use [2].
    (c) The potential for an unrealistic hope of benefit and difficulties in adequately grasping the extent of possible risks should be given special concern when enrolling seriously ill patients [2].

3) *Establishing patient advisory boards, consent monitors, patient advocates,* and other procedures that will concentrate attention on the interests of patient-subjects and their families as these first human trials go forward [2].
4) *Establishing administrative policies* to ensure minimum standards of quality for emerging products before human clinical trials, to enforce consistent reporting requirements for private and public cellular research, to minimize financial conflicts of interest [3].
5) *Conducting much more research* to understand the basic science of the regulation mechanisms of embryonic stem cells, as studies have shown that initial lessons learned on mouse studies may not translate into human embryonic stem cells [44].
6) *Adopting a long-term plan that anticipates problems and prepares for failure and subsequent analysis but ultimately guarantees success.* Scientists must understand that although the current data on transplantation of rodent and human stem cells in animal models is very exciting and demonstrates proof-of-concept, it is not sufficient to enter clinical trials without preparing for setbacks and failures [36].
7) *Considering whom the applications of embryonic stem cells in regenerative medicine would benefit and at what cost,* as well as considering whether these benefits are really worth their price within a national and global health-perspective [23].

8) *Addressing false expectation of a miracle cure through policy issues* to minimize risks for patients as new technologies develop [3].
9) *Being vigilant and flexible to be able to respond to challenges.* The challenge lies in identifying the issues unique to cellular therapy research and incorporating solutions to these challenges into administrative policies to allow forward progress while ultimately preserving patient safety [3].
10) *Encouraging close interaction between basic scientists and clinicians* when developing roadmaps defining the critical steps for each disease, since it is often difficult to reach a consensus in the scientific community when deciding what needs to be done before clinical application.

It can be expected that taking these steps might facilitate the procedure of determining the conditions under which it would be ethically acceptable to proceed with human experimentation.

Acknowledgments

This work was supported by the EU project LHSBCT-2003-503005 (EURO-STEMCELL).

References

[1] The European Association for Bioindustries. Biotech Fact Sheet [cited 2007 Jan 5]. Available from: URL: http://www.europabio.org/documents/tissues-cells.pdf

[2] Dawson L, Bateman-House AS, Mueller Agnew D, Bok H, Brock DW, Chakravarti A et al. Safety issues in cell-based intervention trials. *Fertility and Sterility* 2003; 80: 1077-1085.

[3] Yim R. Administrative and research policies required to bring cellular therapies from the research laboratory to the patient's bedside. *Transfusion* 2005; 45: 144S-158S.

[4] Hawthorne F. Have Stem Cells Finally Arrived? *Chief Executive* 2006; 216: 26-31.

[5] Stipp D. Stem Cells to Fix the Heart. *Fortune* 2004; 150: 179-184.

[6] World Medical Association. Declaration of Helsinki. Ethical Principles for Medical Research Involving Human Subjects. 9.10.2004. [Cited 2007 Jan 3]. Available from: URL: http://www.wma.net/e/policy/b3.htm

[7] Official Journal of the European Communities L 121/34. Directive 2001/20/EC of the European Parliament and of the Council of 4 April 2001 on the approximation of the laws, regulations and administrative provisions of the Member States relating to the implementation of good clinical practice in the conduct of clinical trials on medicinal products for human use. [Cited 2007 Jan 3]. Available from: URL: http://www.esf.org/sciencepolicy /141/Directive.pdf

[8] Commission of the European Communities. Brussels, 16.11.2005. COM (2005) 567 final. 2005/0227 (COD). Proposal for a Regulation of the European Parliament and of the Council on advanced therapy medicinal products and amending Directive

2001/83/EC and Regulation (EC) No 726/2004. [Cited 2007 Jan 3]. Available from: URL:http://ec.europa.eu/enterprise/pharmaceuticals/advtherapies/docs/com_2005_567_en.pdf
[9] Council for International Organizations of Medical Sciences (CIOMS). International Ethical Guidelines for Biomedical Research Involving Human Subjects. Prepared by the Council for International Organizations of Medical Sciences (CIOMS) in collaboration with the World Health Organization (WHO). Geneva 2002. [Cited 2007 Jan 3]. Available from: URL: http://www.cioms. ch/frame_guidelines_nov_2002.htm
[10] Official Journal of the European Union L102/48. Directive 2004/23/EC of the European Parliament and of the Council of 31 March 2004 on setting standards of quality and safety for the donation, procurement, testing, processing, preservation, storage and distribution of human tissues and cells. [Cited 2007 Jan 5]. Available from: URL: http://europa.eu.int/eur-lex/pri/en/oj/dat/2004/l_102/l_10220040407en0048 0058.pdf
[11] Winkler J, Hescheler J, Sachinidis A. Embryonic stem cells for basic research and potential clinical applications in cardiology. *Biochimica et Biophysica Acta (BBA) - Molecular Basis of Disease* 2005; 1740: 240-248.
[12] Lazic SE, Barker RA. The Future of Cell-Based Transplantation Therapies for Neurodegenerative Disorders. *Journal of Hematotherapy and Stem Cell Research* 2003; 12: 635-642.
[13] Reyftmann L, Dechaud H, Hamamah S, Puceat M, Hedon B. Cellules souches embryonnaires : une place pour le gynecologue-obstetricien. Premiere partie. (Embryonic stem cells: A place for an obstetrician-gynaecologist. First part.) *Gynecologie Obstetrique and Fertilite* 2004, 32: 866-871.
[14] Reubinoff B. Human embryonic stem cells - potential applications for regenerative medicine. *International Congress Series* 2004; 1266: 45-53.
[15] Hyslop LA, Armstrong L, Stojkovic M, Lako M. Human embryonic stem cells: biology and clinical implications. *Expert reviews in molecular medicine* 2005; 7: 1-21.
[16] Westendorp RG. Are we becoming less disposable? EMBO Reports 2004; 5: 2-6.
[17] Grusby MJ, Auchincloss H, Lee R, Johnson RS, Spencer JP, Zijlstra M et al. Mice lacking major histocompatibility complex class I and class II molecules. *Proceedings of the National Academy of Sciences of the United States of America* 1993; 90: 3913-3917.
[18] Hochedlinger K, Jaenisch R. Nuclear transplantation, embryonic stem cells, and the potential for cell therapy. *New England journal of medicine* 2003; 349: 275-286.
[19] Munsie MJ, Michalska AE, O'Brien CM, Trounson AO, Pera MF, Mountford PS. Isolation of pluripotent embryonic stem cells from reprogrammed adult mouse somatic cell nuclei. *Current Biology* 2000; 10: 989-992.
[20] Hwang WS, Ryu YJ, Park JH, Park ES, Lee EG, Koo JM et al. Evidence of a pluripotent human embryonic stem cell line derived from a cloned blastocyst. *Science* 2004; 303: 1669-1674.
[21] Cibelli JB, Grant KA, Chapman KB, Cunniff K, Worst T, Green HL et al. Parthenogenetic stem cells in nonhuman primates. *Science* 2002; 295: 819.
[22] Rippon HJ, Bishop AE. Review. Embryonic stem cells. *Cell proliferation* 2004; 37: 23-34.
[23] Borge OJ, Evers K. Aspects on properties, use and ethical considerations of embryonic stem cells – A short review. *Cytotechnology* 2003; 41: 59-68.

[24] Drukker M, Benvenisty N. The immunogenicity of human embryonic stem-derived cells. *Trends in Biotechnology* 2004; 22: 136-141.

[25] Fairchild PJ, Cartland S, Nolan KF, Waldmann H. Embryonic stem cells and the challenge of transplantation tolerance. *Trends in Immun*ology 2004; 25: 465-470.

[26] Parr MJ, Wen PY, Schaub M, Khoury SJ, Sayegh MH, Fine HA. Immune parameters affecting adenoviral vector gene therapy in the brain. *Journal of Neurovirology* 1998; 4: 194-203.

[27] Xiao BG, Link H. Immune regulation within the central nervous system. *Journal of the Neurological Sciences* 1998: 157:1-12.

[28] Reubinoff BE, Pera MF, Fong C-Y, Trounson A, Bongso A. Embryonic stem cell lines from human blastocysts: somatic differentiation in vitro. *Nature Biotechnology* 2000; 18: 399-404.

[29] Schwetz BA. Acting Principal Deputy Commissioner. Letter on Stem Cells to Senator Kennedy. Department of Public Health, U.S. Food and Drug Administration, 5 September 2001. [Cited 2007 Jan 5]. Available from: URL: http://www.fda.gov/oc/stemcells/kennedyltr.html.

[30] Center for Biologics Evaluation and Research. Xenotransplantation action plan: FDA approach to the regulation of xenotransplantation. Center for Biologics Evaluation and Research, U.S. Food and Drug Administration, 17 December 2001. [Cited 2007 Jan 5]. Available from: URL: http://www.fda.gov/cber/xap/xap.htm.

[31] Pedersen RA. Feeding hungry stem cells. *Nature Biotechnology* 2002; 20: 882-3.

[32] Cheng L, Hammond H, Ye Z, Zhan X, Dravid G. Human adult marrow cells support prolonged expansion of human embryonic stem cells in culture. *Stem Cells* 2003; 21: 131-42.

[33] Xu C, Inokuma MS, Denham J, Golds K, Kundu P, Gold JD et al. Feeder-free growth of undifferentiated human embryonic stem cells. *Nature Biotechnology* 2001; 19: 971-974.

[34] Richards M, Fong C-Y, Chan W-K, Wong P-C, Bongso A. Human feeders support prolonged undifferentiated growth of human inner cell masses and embryonic stem cells. *Nature Biotechnology* 2002; 20: 933-936.

[35] Amit M, Margulets V, Segev H, Shariki K, Laevsky I, Coleman R et al. Human feeder layers for human embryonic stem cells. *Biology of Rep*roduction 2003; 68: 2150-2156.

[36] Ginis I, Rao MS. Toward cell replacement therapy: promises and caveats. *Experimental Neurology* 2003; 184: 61-77.

[37] International Conference on Harmonisation of Technical Requirements for Registration of Pharmaceuticals for Human Use. ICH Harmonised Tripartite Guideline. Duration of Chronic Toxicity Testing in Animals (Rodent and Non-Rodent Toxicity Testing). Curent Step 4 version dated 2 September 1998. This Guideline has been developed by the appropriate ICH Expert Working Group and has been subject to consultation by the regulatory parties, in accordance with the ICH Process. At Step 4 of the Process the final draft is recommended for adoption to the regulatory bodies of the European Union, Japan and USA. [Cited 2007 Jan 5]. Available from: URL: http://www.ich.org/LOB/media/MEDIA497.pdf

[38] Corrigan O, Liddell K, McMillan J, Stewart A, Wallace S. Ethical, legal and social issues in stem cell research and therapy. A briefing paper from Cambridge Genetics

Knowledge Park. [Cited 2007 Jan 5]. Available from: URL: http://www.eescn.org.uk/pdfs/elsi_paper.pdf

[39] Dekkers W, Boer G. Sham neurosurgery in patients with Parkinson's disease: is it morally acceptable? *Journal of Medical Ethics* 2001; 27: 151-156.

[40] Weijer C. I need a placebo like I need a hole in the head. *The Journal of law, medicine and ethics: a journal of the American Society of Law, Medicine and Ethics* 2002; 30: 69-72.

[41] Freed CR, Greene PE, Breeze RE, Tsai WY, DuMouchel W, Kao R et al. Transplantation of embryonic dopamine neurons for severe Parkinson's disease. *The New England journal of medicine* 2001; 344: 710-9.

[42] Shalala D. Protecting research subjects - what must be done. The New England journal of medicine 2000; 343: 808-10.

[43] Press releases of the European Commission. Advanced therapies: breakthrough in treating cancer or burned skin. Brussels, 16 November 2005, MEMO/05/429. [Cited 2007 Jan 5]. Available from: URL: http://europa.eu/rapid/ pressReleasesAction.do?reference=MEMO/ 05/429andtype=HTMLandaged=0andlanguage=ENandguiLanguage=en

[44] Sylvester K, Longaker M. Stem cells: review and update. *Archives of Surgery* 2004; 139: 93-9.

In: Stem Cell Therapy and Uses in Medical Treatment
Editor: Prasad S. Koka, pp. 23-34
ISBN: 978-1-61324-008-3

Chapter 2

Survival and Differentiation of Syngeneic Bone Marrow-Derived Mononuclear Cells in Rat Intervertebral Discs

***Helena Brisby**[*1,3]**, Ai-Yun Wei**[1]**, Sylvia Chung**[1]**, Helen Tao**[2]**, David Ma**[2] **and Ashish Diwan**[1]*

[1]Department of Orthopaedic Surgery, St George Hospital, University of New South Wales, Sydney, Australia
[2]Department of Hematology, St Vincent Hospital, University of New South Wales, Sydney, Australia
[3]Department of Orthopedic Surgery, Sahlgrenska University Hospital, Göteborg University, Göteborg, Sweden

Abstract

Main problem: Disc degeneration is characterized by dysfunctional cells and a decrease in extra-cellular components. Transplantation of stem cells and progenitor cells may provide a new approach to treat disc degeneration. In this study we investigate the possibility for stem cells and progenitor cells to survive and differentiate in the non-vascularized intervertebral disc.

Methods: Bone marrow was collected from Sprague-Dawley rats and mononuclear cells isolated. The cells were labeled with a fluorescence dye and transplanted into coccygeal discs in syngeneic rats. Non-injected adjacent discs served as controls. After different time-points (0, 7, 14 or 21 days) the discs were fixed for routine histological staining or processed for cryosections where the number of fluorescein-labeled

* Corresponding author: Helena Brisby, Dept. of Orthopaedics, Sahlgrenska University Hospital, SE413 45 Göteborg Sweden, Fax: +46 31 342 2630. Phone: +46 31 342 10 00; E-mail: helena.brisby@vgregion.se.

transplanted cells was counted. Expression of collagen II was assessed using immunofluorescence technique.

Results: All cell-suspension injected discs contained transplanted bone-marrow cells. There was a decrease in detected cells at 7, 14 and 21 days compared to day 0. Transplanted cells expressed collagen II after 21 days but not after 7 and 14 days.

Conclusions: The results suggest that transplanted bone marrow-derived mononuclear cells can survive and differentiate within the intervertebral disc. Further studies in models of disc degeneration are warranted to investigate the regenerative potential of the disc following cell transplantation.

Keywords: Intervertebral disc, bone marrow derived stem cells, cell transplantation, cell differentiation, disc regeneration.

Introduction

In patients suffering from chronic low back pain, degeneration of the intervertebral disc is clinically considered to be a source of pain[1-5]. The intervertebral disc has a unique structure, composed of two major regions: an outer ring called the annulus fibrosis (AF) and an inner part, nucleus pulposus (NP), with a transitional zone that merges these two regions together. The annulus fibrosis is densely packed with rings composed by fibroblast-like cells and collagen type I. The nucleus pulpous is a gelatinous structure, containing chondrocyte-like cells with proteoglycans and collagen type II. Viable cellular components and balanced surrounding matrix keep the intervertebral discs in shape and maintain normal function.

Disc degeneration may be a sequel to injuries and/or incompetence of the disc tissue to bear normal load. Disc degeneration is characterized by dysfunctional cells and a decrease in extra-cellular components [6, 7]. Cells within the nucleus pulposus express cartilage specific matrix proteins but compared to cartilage chondrocytes there are quantitative differences in expression [8].

Biological methods to regenerate or decelerate the degenerative process may potentially target early disc degeneration and subsequently influence the pain. Theoretically this can be performed by introducing molecules or genes, essential for the regenerative process, into the intervertebral disc where they can influence existing cells [9]. Another way of bio-regeneration of an intervertebral disc could be transplantation of cells from an autologous disc, cartilage or transplantation of immature cells (stem or progenitor cells) which can start to produce new extracellular matrix and thereby reverse the degenerative process.

Cell transplantation to intervertebral discs was first reported by Okuma et al in 2000 [10] using co-cultured annulus fibrosus and nucleus pulposus cells. This concept have also been investigated with autologous or allogeneic disc cells [11-13]. The studies have demonstrated that disc cell therapy delays disc degeneration. Cells from the auricular cartilage have also been transplanted [14] to the intervertebral disc in a rabbit model and a significant percentage of the implanted chondrocytes survived and produced hyaline-like cartilage.

Bone marrow (BM) mononuclear cells contains a subpopulation of cells capable to differentiate to a variety of non-haematopoietic cells [15-17]. These cells are referred to as bone marrow stromal stem cells, multipotent adult progenitor cells or mesenchymal stem cells

(MSC) [18, 19]. Under appropriate experimental conditions, MSCs have been demonstrated to differentiate into specialized cell types of different germ layers such as osteoblasts, adipocytes, chondrocytes, hepatocytes, cardiomyocytes and neural cells [20].

Studies have demonstrated that BM MSCs are able to differentiate into chondrocytes and osteoblasts. These chondrocytic cells express detectable chondrogenic genes and proteins [21] and form cartilage *in vitro* [22]. These interesting findings provide evidence for the possibility of using BM MSCs to heal damaged tissues or treat degenerative diseases. For example, a recent clinical trial addressed the safety, feasibility and demonstrated histological improvement of knee cartilage defects using cultured autologous bone marrow cells for the repair in patients with osteoarthritis [23].

The aim of the present study was to investigate the feasibility of syngeneic bone marrow-derived mononuclear cell transplantation into intervertebral discs in a rat model and to explore if the injected cells start to differentiate towards a disc cell phenotype.

Material and Methods

Isolation and Labelling of BMC

Bone marrow was harvested from femurs and tibia of adult Sprague Dawley rats. Mononuclears cells were isolated by density gradient centrifugation. Briefly, bone marrow cells were fractionated over a 1.077 g/Ficoll-Hypaque solution (Pharmacia, Sweden). Mononuclear cells collected at the interface were suspended in Ca^{++} and Mg^{++} free phosphate buffer saline (PBS) (GIBCO, Invitrogen Life Technologies) at a density of $4x10^7$ and thereafter labelled with 25 μM Cell Tracker Orange (CTO), (Molecular Probes, Eugene, OR) at 37°C for 15 min. The labelled cells were incubated with pre-warmed PBS and centrifuged twice to wash off free dye. For cell transplantation, single cell suspension were prepared in PBS at a concentration of $1x10^7$/ml and stored at 4°C until use.

Intervertebral Disc Transplantation and Specimen Preparation

Sprague–Dawley rats (n=24) with body weight 350-400g were used for mononuclear cell transplantation to the disc. Anaesthesia was achieved by intraperitoneal injection of 80 mg/kg Ketamine and 5mg/kg Xylazine. The intervertebral disc cell transplantation procedures were performed with a 30 gauge needle under sterile condition and fluoroscopic guidance. 10-20μl of cells in PBS suspension ($1x10^7$ cells /ml) was injected in each disc. Two discs for each animal were injected and one disc served as control.

Animals were euthanized at day 0, day 7 and day 21 post injection and spinal column specimens were collected. The disc and vertebrae were fixed immediately with 10% neutral buffered formalin for 24 hours. For cell counting and immunofluorescence staining tissues were placed in tissue freezing medium, rapidly frozen in liquid nitrogen and stored at -80°C until processed. For histology the tissues were placed in RDO solution (rapid decalcification reagent) for 36 hours after fixation in formalin.

Cell Culture

Fluorescent labelled MNCs were grown in Dulbecco's modified Eagle's medium (DMEM) (GIBCO, Invitrogen Life Technologies) with 4.5% of glucose, supplemented with 10% of fetal bovine serum (FBS) and 100 IU/ml of penicillin plus 100 μg/ml of streptomycin.

All cells were maintained in 25 cm^2 flasks at 37°C in 100% humidity atmosphere and 5% of CO_2. Medium was changed every 3-5 days. OCT labelled cells was detected with inverted fluorescence microscopy.

Histology

After fixation and decalcification the tissue was dehydrated and embedded in paraffin. Mid-sagittal sections was cut at 5μm thickness and stained with hematoxyline/eosin (HandE) and alcian blue. The stained sections were examined with a Lecia DMLB microscope (Leica, Germany), disc height and gross morphological assessment performed.

Cell Counting

Cryosections were obtained in the transverse plane, approximately 8 μm thick and dried at room temperature for 30 min. For each disc 25 to 40 sections were cut. Ten complete disc sections without folds on the slide glass were chosen; these sections represented the upper, middle and lower part of the disc. The sections were counter stained with DAPI (4',6-Diamidino-2-phenylindole dihydrochloride, Sigma Aldrich, St Louis MO, USA) to visualize the cells in the tissue. To determine the number of cells labelled with CTO in vitro, the total number of labelled cells was counted using a 20X objective in the 10 macroscopically selected sections. The cell counts were assessed by two investigators blinded to the source of the tissue.

Immune Fluorescence Staining

A collagen II rabbit polyclonal antibody (Chemicon International, Australia) was used to detect cells expressing collagen II. Frozen 8 μm thick sections were fixed in ice-cold acetone for 15 minutes, and dried at room temperature. Non-specific antigens were savaged by 5% normal goat serum, thereafter the tissue sections were incubated with collagen type II antibody (1:100) for 2 hours at room temperature. After washing, the sections were treated with FITC-conjugated goat-anti-rabbit immunoglobulin (Chemicon International). Sections were mounted with non-fluorescent anti-fade medium (DAKO) for visualisation. In order to subtract background autofluorescence, negative controls were treated according to the same protocol with the omission of primary antibody and were consistently included in each experiment. The fluorescence positive cells in tissue sections were assessed by two investigators blinded to the source of tissue.

Ethics

The study was approved by the Animal Care and Ethics Committee of University of New South Wales, Sydney, and performed in accordance with the committee's regulations.

Statistical Analyses

Numbers of cells are expressed as mean ± standard error of the mean (SEM). The non-parametric Kruskal-Wallis test followed by Mann Whitney's test was used to compare number of cells at different time points.

Results

Cell Culture

Bone marrow mononuclear cells labelled with fluorescent dye (OCT) maintained their fluorescence when kept in cell culture for three weeks. During the three-week time period the cells proliferated and the daughter cells were also fluorescent (Figure 1).

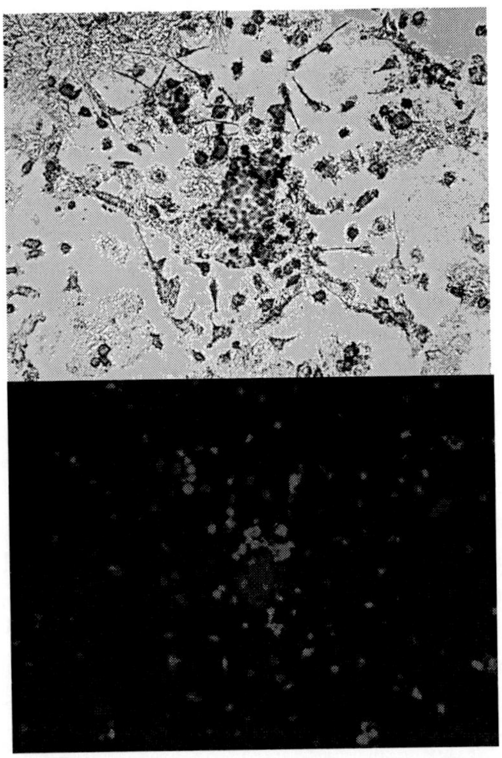

Figure 1. Cultured bone marrow derived mononuclear cells remained fluorescent at 21 days (100x).

Histology

No changes in disc height, cell or matrix formation could be seen in the cell transplanted discs compared to the control discs (Figure 2). No signs of inflammatory reactions within or around the discs were seen.

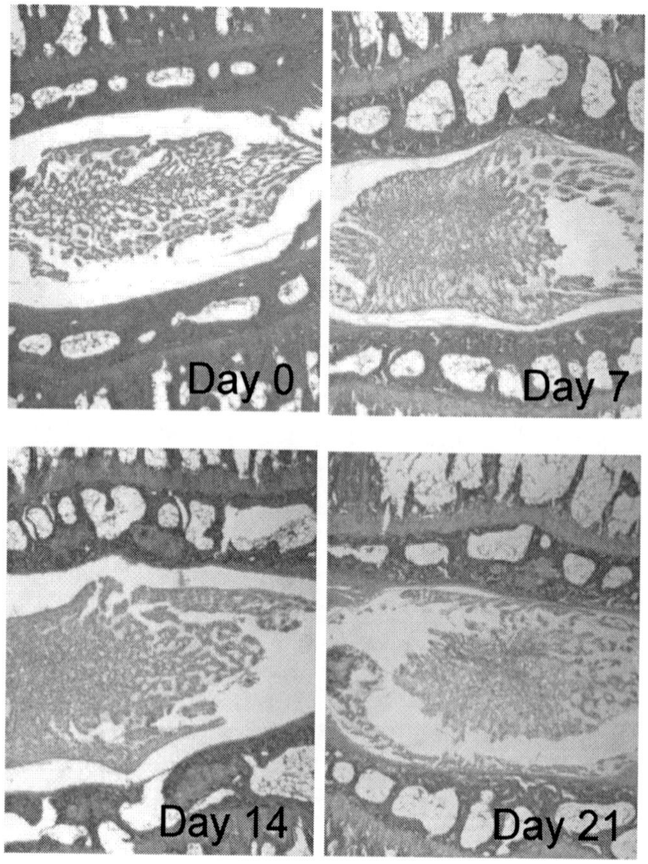

Figure 2. No histological changes could be seen in the discs at any time points after transplantation of bone-marrow derived mononuclear cells.

Number of Cells

All cell-suspension injected discs contained transplanted bone-marrow cells (Figure 3).

The discs within each time-group demonstrated a large variation in the number of transplanted cells detected. There was a significant difference between the number of detected cells at the different time-points ($p<0.0001$, Kruskal-Wallis test). There were a decrease in detected cells at 7, 14 and 21 days compared to baseline (day 0), a statistical decrease between day 7 and 14 but no statistically significant differences between the two latter time points (Figure 4). The cells were unevenly distributed within the whole nucleus pulposus of the disc (Figure 5). Only a few cells were detected in the annulus fibrosus. No positive cells could be detected in any of the control discs.

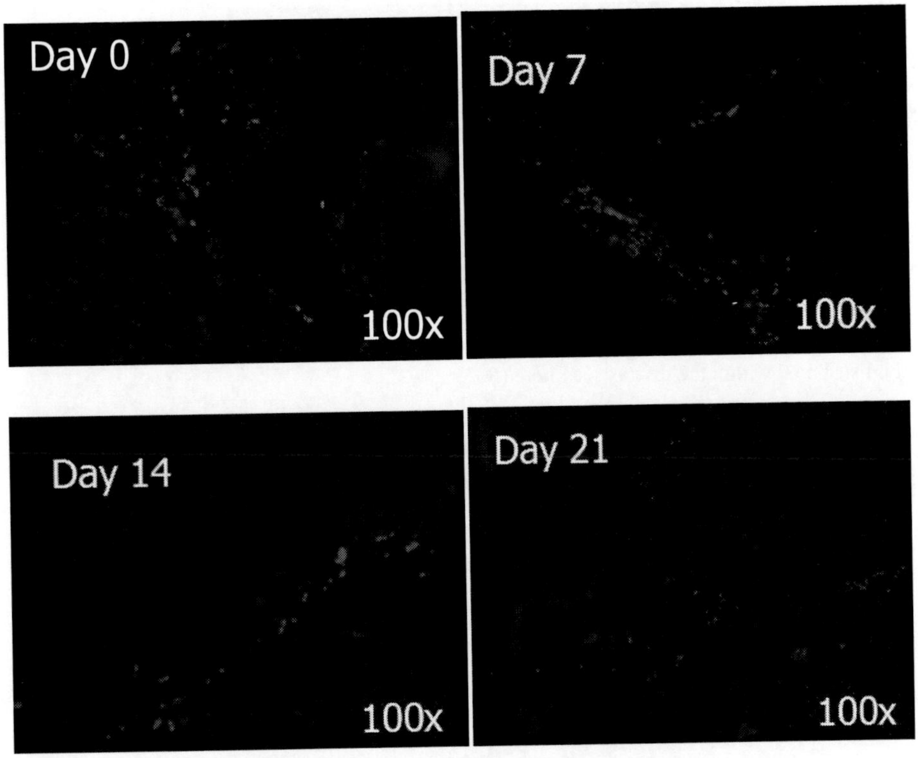

Figure 3. The transplanted bone-marrow derived mononuclear cells were detected within the intervertebral discs at all investigated timepoints.

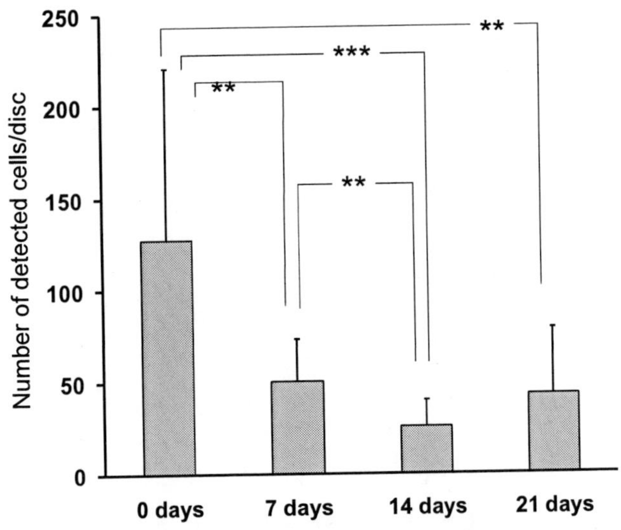

Figure 4. Number of transplanted cells/section at different time-points. 10 discs were investigated at each time point and the cells counted in ten sections per disc. There was a significant difference between the number of detected cells at the different time-points ($p<0.0001$ Kruskal-Wallis test). A decrease of detected cells was seen soon after transplantation (compare day 0 and day 7). The number of detected cells at day 14 after transplantation significantly decreased compared to day 0 and day 7. No difference was observed between day 14 and 21.

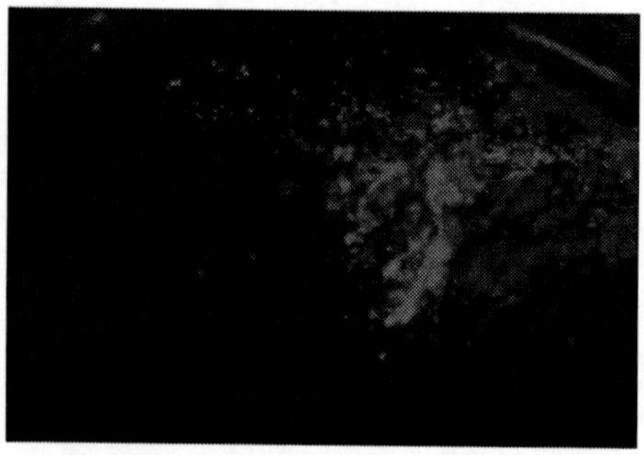

Figure 5. The transplanted cells were mainly detected within the nucleus pulposus of the disc and often unevenly distributed within the disc as seen here (50X).

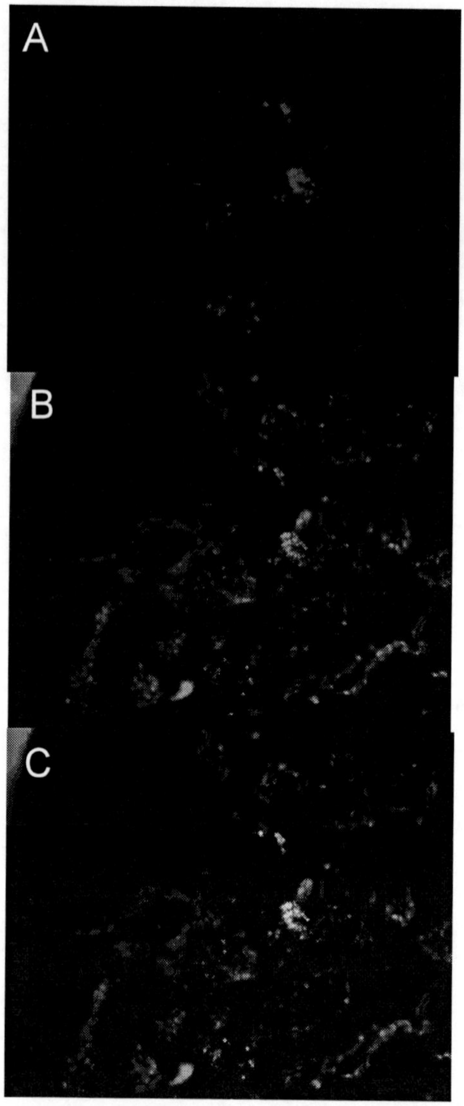

Figure 6. Transplanted mononuclear cells expressed collagen II (green) at 21 days post transplantation (100x). A) transplanted cells (red), B) Collagen II staining cells/tissue (green), C) A and B merged. No transplanted cells expressed collagen II at the earlier timepoints (not shown in the picture).

Cell Differentiation

Aproximately 30 % of the transplanted cells were positive for type II collagen staining at 21 days (Figure 6).

No transplanted cells expressed type II collagen at day 0, 7 or 14 days. Labelled BM MNC cells kept in culture did not express type II collagen at any time point up to 21 days.

Discussion

The present study demonstrates that syngeneic bone marrow derived mononuclear cells survive after transplantation into intervertebral discs. Further, the results suggest that the transplanted cells start to differentiate towards disc cells by 21 days post transplantation.

The present study was limited to 21 days post-transplantation and we found that the transplanted cells survived the study period. However, the number of transplanted cells decreased by 60-70 % at day 7 and 14 post-transplantation; and then tended to increase at day 21, (Figure 1). This suggests that the majority of the transplanted cells died during the first 2 weeks after transplantation and that the surviving cells possibly start to proliferate within weeks. Our results are similar to those reported by Crevenstern et al's study where mesenchymal stem cells were transplanted with hyaluronan as a carrier [24]. These authors demonstrated a decrease in number of cells at day 7 and 14 but observed a statistically insignificant increase in number of cells at day 28. In both these studies unsorted bone-marrow derived mononuclear cells containing non-haematopoietic stem cells, i.e. mesenchymal stem cells, were used. These stem cells have been established to have the ability to contribute to the generation of non-haematopoietic tissues. However, the optimal cell population for regeneration of different organ system remains to be established. The differentiated cells within the unsorted mononuclear cell population used might be part of the reason for the rapid decrease in detectable cells after disc transplantation. The poor nutrition of the disc and the low pH also are factors which may contribute to rapid cell loss after transplantation.

In the study reported by Sakai et al, bone marrow-derived mesenchymal stem cells were tested in a disc-degeneration rabbit model [25]. In this study an increase in disc height and proteoglycan content following cell transplantation was demonstrated. The transplanted cells in this study were embedded into a carrier (Atelocollagen) and the study did not isolate the effect of the cells or carrier alone. In the present study, cells were implanted into healthy, non-degenerated disc to study cell survival and as the normal supportive matrix in the disc was present for the implanted cells, no carrier was needed. However, cells transplanted into a degenerated disc may require a carrier to provide a structural and nutritional support for the transplanted cells. Another possible reason to use a carrier could be to ensure delivery of cells by injection to the disc since the intradiscal pressure and gelatinous structure have been suggested to be less favourable for injection of a suspension [26]. Interestingly in the present study we found that the cells were widely spread out within the disc when transplanted in suspension.

The finding of collagen II-expressing transplanted cells at day 21 after injection indicates that a subpopulation of the cells not only survived in the disc, but also adapted and responded to the microenvironment. This study supports Sakai et al's work by demonstrating that the transplanted cells can potentially increase the extracellular matrix secretion.

The therapeutic potential of adult stem cells for autologous regeneration of the intervertebral disc is a new area. The present study was limited by a relatively short observation time. However, the findings in this study confirm previous observations that it is feasible to transplant bone-marrow derived cells to the intervertebral disc, and demonstrated for the first time that this can be achieved without using a carrier. Further, some transplanted cells changed their phenotype and expressed collagen II within 21 days. These findings encourage further work to explore stem cell therapy for the regeneration of the intervertebral disc.

Conclusion

- Bone marrow-derived mononuclear cells (BMC´s) can survive up to 21 days after transplantation to the intervertebral disc in a rat model.
- It is feasible to transplant BMC´s to the intervertebral disc without using a carrier.
- Transplanted cells express collagen type II 21 days after transplantation to the intervertebral disc.

Acknowledgments

This study was supported by Gothenburg Medical Association, Nordic Orthopaedic Federation (Göran Bauer´s Grant), Swedish Medical Association, Wennergren foundation, International Society for Study of the Lumbar Spine (ISSLS), Spine Service St George Hospital Campus Sydney, South East Health, Sydney, and St Vincent's Hospital Sydney Haematology Research Fund.

References

[1] Lee, K.S., et al., Diagnostic criteria for the clinical syndrome of internal disc disruption: are they reliable? *Br. J. Neurosurg*, 2003. 17(1): p. 19-23.

[2] Paajanen, H., et al., Age-dependent correlation of low-back pain and lumbar disc regeneration. *Arch. Orthop. Trauma Surg.*, 1997. 116(1-2): p. 106-7.

[3] Peterson, C.K., J.E. Bolton, and A.R. Wood, A cross-sectional study correlating lumbar spine degeneration with disability and pain. *Spine*, 2000. 25(2): p. 218-23.

[4] Ito, M., et al., Predictive signs of discogenic lumbar pain on magnetic resonance imaging with discography correlation. *Spine*, 1998. 23(11): p. 1252-8; discussion 1259-60.

[5] Elfering, A., et al., Risk factors for lumbar disc degeneration: a 5-year prospective MRI study in asymptomatic individuals. *Spine*, 2002. 27(2): p. 125-34.

[6] Boos, N., et al., Classification of age-related changes in lumbar intervertebral discs: 2002 Volvo Award in basic science. *Spine,* 2002. 27(23): p. 2631-44.
[7] Walker, M.H. and D.G. Anderson, Molecular basis of intervertebral disc degeneration. *Spine J.*, 2004. 4(6 Suppl): p. 158S-166S.
[8] Poiraudeau, S., et al., Phenotypic characteristics of rabbit intervertebral disc cells. Comparison with cartilage cells from the same animals. *Spine*, 1999. 24(9): p. 837-44.
[9] Wallach, C.J., L.G. Gilbertson, and J.D. Kang, Gene therapy applications for intervertebral disc degeneration. *Spine,* 2003. 28(15): p. S93-8.
[10] Okuma, M., et al., Reinsertion of stimulated nucleus pulposus cells retards intervertebral disc degeneration: an in vitro and in vivo experimental study. *J. Orthop. Res.*, 2000. 18(6): p. 988-97.
[11] Watanabe, K., et al., Effect of reinsertion of activated nucleus pulposus on disc degeneration: an experimental study on various types of collagen in degenerative discs. *Connect Tissue Res.*, 2003. 44(2): p. 104-8.
[12] Sato, M., et al., An experimental study of the regeneration of the intervertebral disc with an allograft of cultured annulus fibrosus cells using a tissue-engineering method. *Spine*, 2003. 28(6): p. 548-53.
[13] Nomura, T., et al., Nucleus pulposus allograft retards intervertebral disc degeneration. *Clin. Orthop.*, 2001(389): p. 94-101.
[14] Gorensek, M., et al., Nucleus pulposus repair with cultured autologous elastic cartilage derived chondrocytes. *Cell Mol. Biol. Lett.,* 2004. 9(2): p. 363-73.
[15] Pittenger, M.F., et al., Multilineage potential of adult human mesenchymal stem cells. *Science*, 1999. 284(5411): p. 143-7.
[16] Prockop, D.J., Marrow stromal cells as stem cells for nonhematopoietic tissues. *Science,* 1997. 276(5309): p. 71-4.
[17] Verfaillie, C.M., M.F. Pera, and P.M. Lansdorp, Stem cells: hype and reality. *Hematology* (Am Soc Hematol Educ Program), 2002: p. 369-91.
[18] Short, B., et al., Mesenchymal stem cells. *Arch. Med. Res.*, 2003. 34(6): p. 565-71.
[19] Seshi, B., S. Kumar, and D. Sellers, Human bone marrow stromal cell: coexpression of markers specific for multiple mesenchymal cell lineages. *Blood Cells Mol. Dis.*, 2000. 26(3): p. 234-46.
[20] Tao, H.a.M.D.F., Evidence for transdifferentiation of human bone marrow-derived stem cells: recent progress and controversies. *Pathology*, 2003. 35(1): p. 6-13.
[21] Barry, F., et al., Chondrogenic differentiation of mesenchymal stem cells from bone marrow: differentiation-dependent gene expression of matrix components. *Exp. Cell Res.*, 2001. 268(2): p. 189-200.
[22] Sekiya, I., et al., In vitro cartilage formation by human adult stem cells from bone marrow stroma defines the sequence of cellular and molecular events during chondrogenesis. *Proc. Natl. Acad. Sci. USA*, 2002. 99(7): p. 4397-402.
[23] Wakitani, S., et al., Human autologous culture expanded bone marrow mesenchymal cell transplantation for repair of cartilage defects in osteoarthritic knees. *Osteoarthritis Cartilage*, 2002. 10(3): p. 199-206.
[24] Crevensten, G., et al., Intervertebral disc cell therapy for regeneration: mesenchymal stem cell implantation in rat intervertebral discs. *Ann. Biomed. Eng.*, 2004. 32(3): p. 430-4.

[25] Sakai, D., et al., Transplantation of mesenchymal stem cells embedded in Atelocollagen gel to the intervertebral disc: a potential therapeutic model for disc degeneration. *Biomaterials*, 2003. 24(20): p. 3531-41.

[26] Ananthakrishnan, D., et al. Carrier matrix viscosity influences mesenchymal stem cell delivery to the intervertebral disc. In 49th *Annual Meeting of the Orthopaedic Research Society*. 2003. New Orleans, USA.

In: Stem Cell Therapy and Uses in Medical Treatment
Editor: Prasad S. Koka, pp. 35-64
ISBN: 978-1-61324-008-3

Chapter 3

Current Therapies for Multiple Sclerosis: Stem Cells or Immunomodulators?

Masha Fridkis-Hareli*
Department of Cancer Immunology and AIDS,
Dana Farber Cancer Institute, and Department of Pathology,
Harvard Medical School, Boston, MA, USA

Abstract

During the past decade, major advances in the treatment of multiple sclerosis (MS) have been accomplished mainly due to the introduction of immunomodulatory and immunosuppressive agents, which have significantly altered the natural course of this incurable and disabling neurodegenerative disorder. Recent studies have demonstrated the importance of the early initiation of treatment for the reduction of short-term and potentially long-term neurological impairment associated with MS. However, despite early diagnosis and early initiation of therapy, patients still experience breakthrough relapses and progression of their underlying MS pathology. The imperfect effectiveness, side effects, and toxicity of these agents, emphasize the necessity for development of more effective medications with less adverse events. It is increasingly recognized that MS progression, in addition to demyelination, leads to substantial irreversible damage to, and loss of neurons, resulting in brain atrophy and cumulative disability. One of the most promising neuroprotective strategies involves the use of bone marrow (BM) derived stem cells. Both hematopoietic and non-hematopoietic (stromal) cells can, under certain circumstances, differentiate into cells of various neuronal and glial lineages. Consequently, stem cell transplantation has been increasingly considered for the therapy-resistant MS. In this review, the status of the current therapies for MS is discussed in the

* Corresponding author: Masha Fridkis-Hareli, Ph.D., Department of Cancer Immunology and AIDS, Dana Farber Cancer Institute, 44 Binney St, Boston, MA, 02115. Phone (617)632-3344, Fax (617)632-4468, email: masha_fridkis-hareli@dfci.harvard.edu

context of long-term remission benefits as relates to the mechanisms of immunopathology and immunoregulation. The outcome of ongoing clinical trials, as well as of studies in patients and animal models, will help to determine the role of stem-cell transplantation in the treatment of MS. Furthermore, it seems that future therapeutic strategies for MS should combine immunomodulation with neuroprotective modalities to achieve maximal clinical benefit.

Keywords: Immunomodulation; multiple sclerosis; stem cell transplantation.

Abbreviations: APC, antigen-presenting cells; BM, bone marrow; GA, glatiramer acetate; HSC, haematopoietic stem cells; MS, multiple sclerosis; PPMS, primary-progressive multiple sclerosis; RRMS, relapsing-remitting multiple sclerosis.

Introduction

Multiple sclerosis (MS) is a chronic autoimmune inflammatory disease of the central nervous system. Damage to the myelin sheath, which coats nerve fibers, interferes with their ability to transmit impulses to each other and to other parts of the body, causing problems with muscle control, coordination, walking, vision, balance, sensation, thinking, and bowel and bladder function. MS is the most common, non-traumatic, neurological disease in young adults, affecting approximately 400,000 Americans and two million people worldwide. Age of onset is typically between 20 and 40 years, and women are more likely to be affected than men. The relapsing-remitting form of MS, characterized by flares interspersed with symptom-free periods for up to 10 years, accounts for about 90% of cases. The remaining 10% are primary progressive, meaning that neurologic impairment and disability continue to worsen. Even in relapsing-remitting MS, however, the exacerbations may not clear completely, and each relapse tends to increase the patient's residual level of disability.

The diagnosis of MS was once approached with the intent to provide symptomatic relief for patients, with little hope of impacting the natural history of their illness. However, the past decade has introduced major advances in the treatment of MS. In the era of immune-omodulatory drugs, there has been a paradigm shift in the approach to MS therapy resulting in a significant change of the disease course. Recent studies have demonstrated that early initiation of treatment may reduce short-term and potentially long-term neurological impairment associated with MS [1-4]. Among disease-modifying drugs approved for treatment of relapsing forms of MS, the three interferon-β preparations (Avonex, Betaseron and Rebif) and glatiramer acetate (Copaxone) serve as first-line agents, and have been in routine use for approximately a decade. These parenteral therapies are not reparative but preventive in action, and reduce MS relapses by one-third [5-10]. Mitoxantrone and nataluzimab are held in reserve as second-line MS therapies for more aggressive forms of the disease due to their potential deleterious side effects [11].

In spite of the apparent success of the immunomodulatory agents in suppressing the immunopathologic manifestations of MS, current treatments are only partially effective, probably due to defective remyelinating-regenerating mechanisms. These include insufficient growth factors and multipotential stem cells [12], resulting in chronic, cumulative disability and irreversible axonal/neuronal damage [13-15]. It has also been suggested that the course of

MS proceeds in two phases, an initial inflammatory and a degenerative one [16, 17]. Hence, different type of therapeutic interventions, in addition to immunomodulation, would be needed in order to improve the treatment outcome in MS. This other set of therapies is aimed at addressing the complicated relationship between the three key pathogenetic elements of MS, inflammation, demyelination and axonal damage. It is well established that inflammation can cause demyelination [18] and both inflammation and myelin destruction can damage the axons, leading to the induction of neurodegeneration [15, 19-21]. Importantly, it is increasingly recognized that certain aspects of inflammation may be beneficial for MS [22], causing neuroprotection via the local production of growth factors [23] or by direct cell to cell interactions with oligodendrocyte progenitors [17].

Whilst many current neuroprotective methods aim to prevent axonal injury, another possibility might be to encourage remyelination; one method by which this may be achieved is by stem cell transplantation. It has been previously shown that neuronal stem cells can suppress experimental allergic encephalomyelitis (EAE, an animal model for MS) by exerting peripheral and in situ immunomodulating effects, in addition to being a possible source for remyelination and neuroregeneration [24-26]. Another potential source for stem cells could be the bone marrow (BM) non-hematopoietic, mesenchymal stromal cells (MSC). These cells can exhibit stem cell features and differentiate, under certain circumstances, into cells of various tissue lineages, including neurons and glia [27, 28]. Therefore, both BM and neuronal stem cells could have therapeutic potential in various neurodegenerative diseases. BM derived MSCs offer practical advantages over conventional embryonic neuronal stem cells: (1) they can easily be obtained from adult BM, (2) they can easily be cultured and expanded and (3) they can be injected autologously without the need for immunosuppression.

The present study is a comprehensive review of the current immunomodulatory therapies for MS including disease-modifying drugs and stem cell transplantation. These approaches are discussed in the context of their long-term remission benefits as related to the mechanisms of immunopathology and immunoregulation. In addition, the rational and the status of ongoing clinical trials in MS patients with novel compounds and combination therapy is presented herewith.

Stem Cell Therapy for MS

Neuronal Stem Cells

Stem cells hold a great therapeutic potential for injury and disease in humans due to their unique ability for both self-renewing and differentiating into many different cell types that make up the organism. With the recent advances in purification and characterization of the tissue-specific stem cells, it now became feasible to isolate them from many tissues of more advanced developmental stages such as BM mesenchymal stem cells, hematopoietic stem cells and neural stem cells. The later have the capacity to grow indefinitely and to differentiate into three major cell types of CNS - neurons, astrocytes and oligodendrocytes [29-31].

It has been increasingly recognized that MS progression, in addition to demyelination, leads to substantial irreversible damage to, and loss of neurons, resulting in brain atrophy and cumulative disability. One of the most promising neuroprotective strategies involves the use of BM-derived stem cells. Both hematopoietic and non-hematopoietic (stromal) cells can, under certain circumstances, differentiate into cells of various neuronal and glial lineages. Neuronal stem cells have also been reported to suppress EAE by exerting direct in situ immunomodulating effects, in addition to their ability to provide a potential source for remyelination and neuroregeneration. Both BM and neuronal stem cells may therefore have a therapeutic potential in MS. While many current neuroprotective methods aim to prevent axonal injury, another possibility might be to encourage remyelination; one method by which this may be achieved is by stem cell transplantation. Neuronal stem cells were shown to suppress EAE by exerting peripheral and in situ immunomodulating effects, in addition to being a possible source for remyelination and neuroregeneration [24-26]. In addition, BM non-hematopoietic, mesenchymal stromal cells (MSC), which exhibit stem cell features and differentiate into cells of various tissue lineages, including neurons and glia, could represent another potential source for stem cells [27, 28].

Myelin-producing oligodendrocyte progenitor cells are found abundantly in the adult human brain [32]. Spontaneous remyelination occurs to varying degrees in the early stages of MS, and these cells are also detected in chronic demyelinated MS lesions. An important area of research is aimed at finding ways to enhance remyelination from these cells, and identifying the factors that lead to a failure of cells to produce myelin in the first place. To this end, Back *et al.* [33] recently showed that astrocyte-derived hyaluronan accumulated in demyelinated lesions from MS patients and prevented the maturation of endogenous oligodendrocyte progenitors. The transplantation of remyelinating cells represents another approach for treating myelin loss in MS. Human adult [22] and ES-cell-derived [34] progenitors have been shown to myelinate dysmyelinated mouse brain and spinal cord after transplantation. However, a major concern is that the inflammatory environment could destroy the grafted oligodendrocyte precursors and inhibit their maturation. Immunosuppressive and anti-inflammatory treatments might therefore be necessary. Another problem is that the demyelinated MS lesions are distributed across multiple locations throughout the CNS. An effective therapy will require the implanted OPCs to migrate to these sites. Interestingly, after systemic administration in mice, NS cells migrated to inflammatory demyelinating lesions, where some became OPCs and remyelinated axons [25]. Most cells remained undifferentiated and suppressed proinflammatory mechanisms [35].

Oligodendrocyte lineage cells can be expanded from various sources, such as neural stem cells from the developing brain, and embryonic stem cells [32]. Following intraventricular transplantation of undifferentiated neurospheres into rodents with EAE, the cells migrate into the inflamed white matter and acquire glial lineages markers. Staining of cells that have been tagged with BrdU prior to transplantation showed their migration in the corpus callosum of EAE animals, while double labeling with GalC indicated that the transplanted cells differentiated into mature oligodendrocytes. Intraventricular transplantation of neurospheres into mice with chronic EAE attenuated the clinical course of the paralytic disease. This was associated with reduction of demyelination and of axonal injury in the cell-transplanted animals compared to sham-transplanted mice [24, 26]. These precursor cells seem to be safely suitable for human transplantation. They may also serve as vectors for the delivery of therapeutic genes and proteins via precursor cells utilizing their capacity for stable integration in the CNS.

In a series of preliminary experiments, the therapeutic potential of BM MSCs in chronic progressive EAE has been tested, using both the unmanipulated and the purified cells [36]. BM SC migrated into the inflamed lesions and showed morphological and immunohistological features indicating differentiation into astrocytes, neuronal and glial cells. The clinical course of EAE was significantly ameliorated in animals treated with BM SC or purified BM SC. Recently, other groups have stressed the therapeutic potential of mouse and human BMSCs in the animal model of MS, EAE, focusing mainly on the immunomodulatory properties of these cells when administered intravenously [37, 38]. In summary, a combined approach of immunomodulation and neuroprotection will be needed in order to improve the therapeutic outcome in MS [39, 40]. Potential applications of neuronal stem cells for the treatment of MS are depicted in Figure 1.

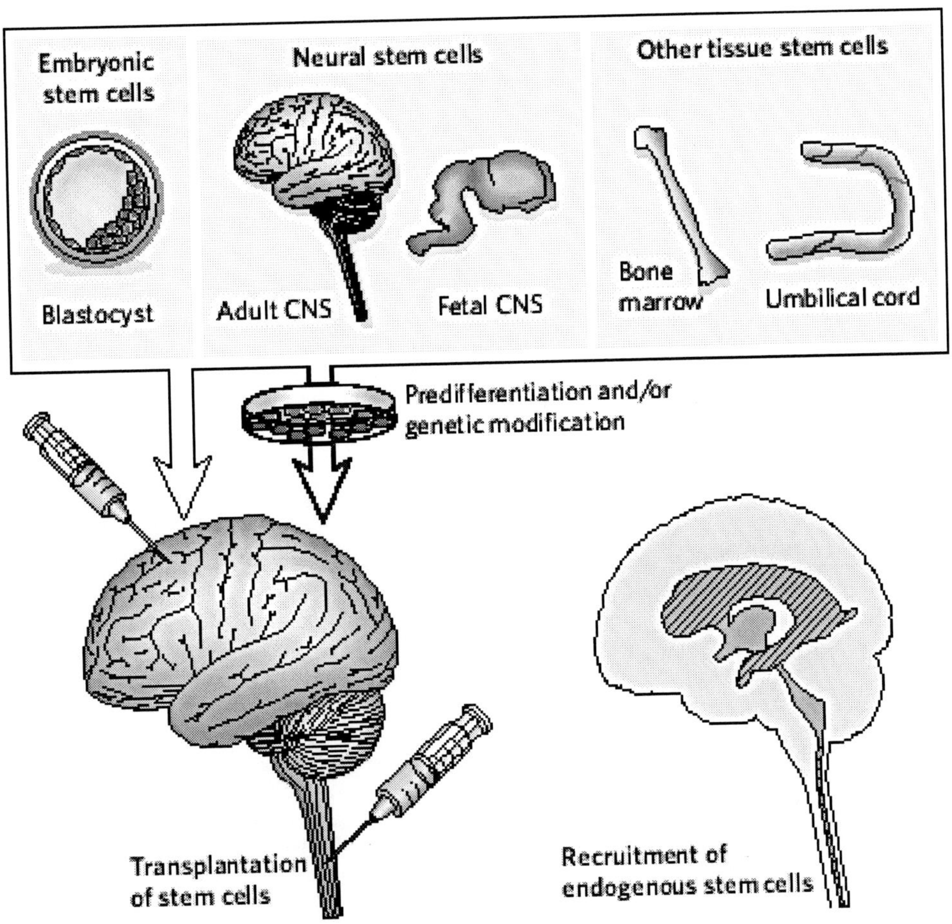

Figure 1. Application of stem cells for neurological disorders. Stem cells would be isolated and transplanted to the diseased brain and spinal cord, either directly or after predifferentiation/genetic modification in culture to form specific types of neuron and glial cell, or cells producing neuroprotective molecules. In strategies relying on stimulation of the patient's own repair mechanisms, endogenous stem cells would be recruited to areas of the adult brain and spinal cord affected by disease, where they would produce new neurons and glia (neurogenic and gliogenic areas along lateral ventricle and central canal are shown in hatched red). Stem cells could provide clinical benefits by neuronal replacement, remyelination and neuroprotection (adopted from ref. [37]).

Bone Marrow-Derived Haematopoietic Stem Cells

While the investigation of the neuroprotective potential of neuronal stem cells for the treatment of MS remains at the initial pre-clinical stages, the use of BM-derived haematopoietic stem cells (HSC) has become increasingly widespread in the immunotherapy-resistant MS cases. Transplantation of HSC involves administration of mobilized peripheral blood cells and BM cells, both of which are enriched for HSC, into the patient, resulting in their self-renewing and differentiation into all mature haematopoietic cell types and possibly some non- haematopoietic cell types. The HSC phenotype is characterized by a lack of cell-surface lineage markers and the expression of CD34 in humans. The inclusion of other cells besides HSC, especially lymphocytes, in the mixture for transplantation, has considerable potential to influence the outcome of the therapy.

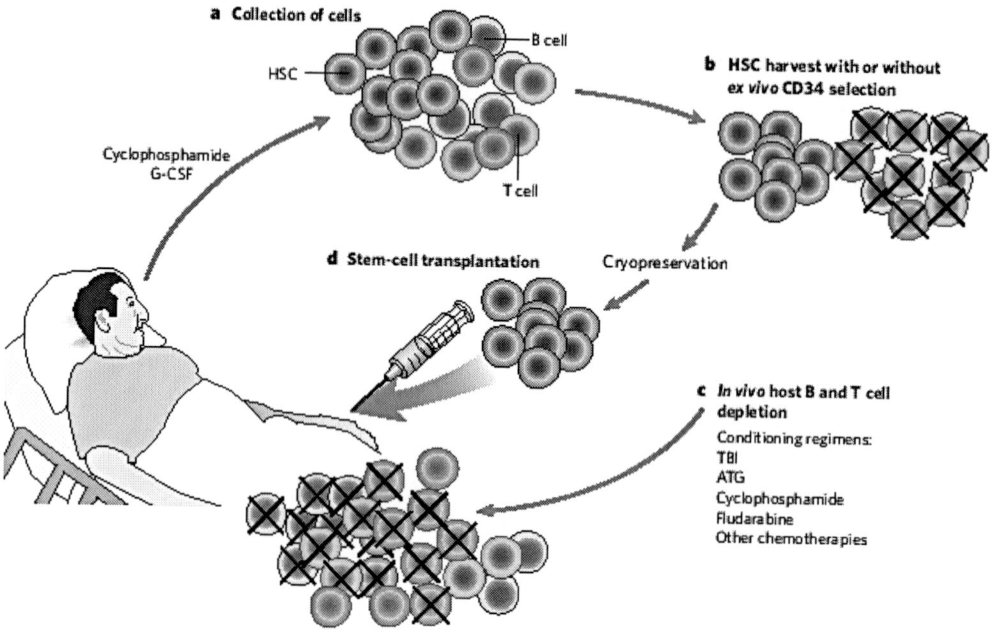

Figure 2. Autologous HCT as a therapy for autoimmune disease. Red cells represent autoreactive host lymphocytes; green cells represent non-autoreactive host lymphocytes; blue cells represent HSC. The steps in autologous HCT include the following. a, Stem-cell collection: HSCs are either harvested from the bone marrow under anaesthesia or collected aftermobilization to the peripheral blood by treating the patient with growth factor (for example, G-CSF) and/or chemotherapy (for example, cyclophosphamide). b, HSC harvest, with or without ex vivo selection using antibody specific for CD34 (a marker of HSCs): efforts may or may not be made to deplete T and B cells from the marrow or mobilized peripheral blood cells. This is usually achieved by HSC positive selection on the basis of CD34 expression. The HSC preparation is cryopreserved. c, In vivo lymphocyte depletion: various conditioning regimens with the goal of minimizing the burden of autoreactive B and T cells are given to patients. These include combinations of chemotherapeutic agents, total-body irradiation (TBI) and in vivo lymphocyte depletion by antibodies, such as anti-thymocyte globulin (ATG), and these treatments often deplete host HSC as well. d, Stem-cell transplantation: after conditioning, the cryopreserved HSC preparation is thawed and returned to the recipient to reconstitute haematopoiesis (adopted from ref. [41]).

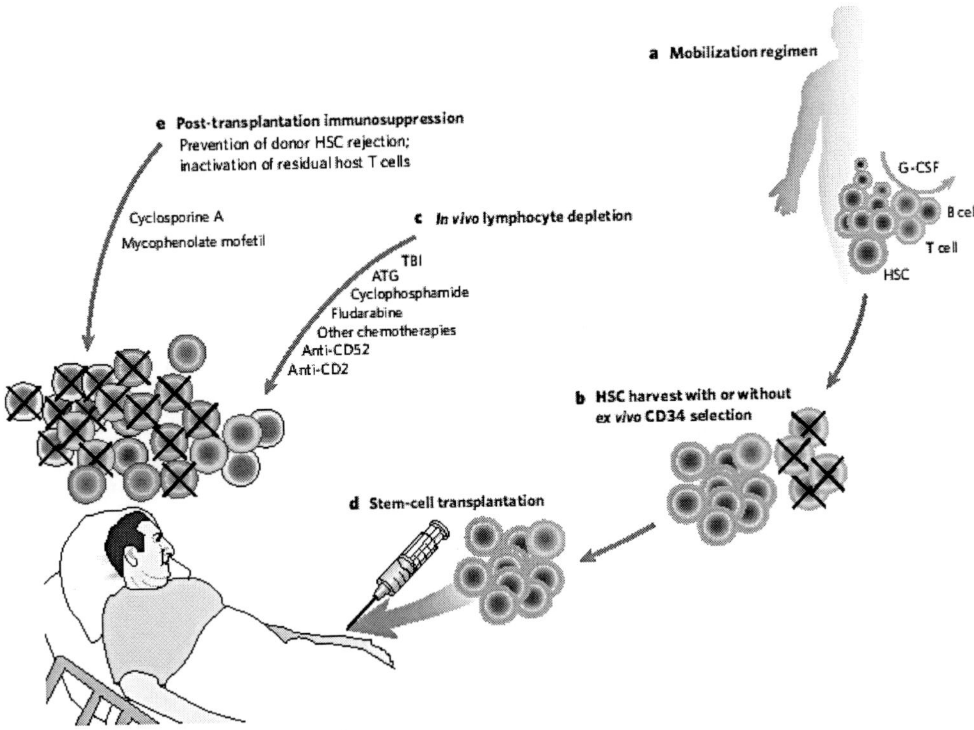

Figure 3. Allogeneic HCT as a therapy for autoimmune disease. Red cells represent autoreactive host lymphocytes; green cells represent non-autoreactive host lymphocytes; yellow denotes donor lymphocytes; blue cells represent HSC. The steps in allogeneic HCT include the following. a, Mobilization regimen: these are similar to the methods employed for autologous HCT, except that cyclophosphamide and other chemotherapies are not used to mobilize stem cells. Mobilization is achieved using the growth factor G-CSF. b, HSC harvest, with or without ex vivo CD34 selection. This step is similar to that used for auto-HCT. c, In vivo lymphocyte depletion: this step depletes host T and B cells to prevent rejection and treat the autoimmune disease; it may also be aimed at depleting donor T cells (to prevent GVHD). d, Stem-cell transplantation: as for auto-HCT. e, Post-transplantation immunosuppression: as prophylaxis against both rejection mediated by residual host T cells and GVHD mediated by contaminating donor T cells, allo-HCT usually requires additional post-transplantation immunosupression with agents such as cyclosporine A and mycophenolate mofetil (adopted from ref. [41]).

The patient is prepared for the transplant by potent immunosuppressive treatment, usually by chemotherapy and/or radiotherapy. This protocol is followed by the transfer of autologous haematopoietic cells (harvested from the patient before conditioning) or allogeneic haematopoietic cells (harvested from donors) to restore the host immune system. This procedure can cure autoimmune disease in experimental animals and is now being explored in human clinical trials. The scheme of the clinical protocol for autologous and allogeneic stem cell transplantation is represented in Figures 2 and 3, respectively. To this end, autologous HSC have been generally preferred over allogeneic HSC because of the increased toxicity and potential for rejection in the later. The risk of the graft-versus-host-disease in the case of allogeneic HSC transplantation, which arises from the attack of donor allogeneic T cells on recipient alloantigens, is associated with significant morbidity and mortality.

Nevertheless, allogeneic HSC transplantation has been associated with durable complete remission in a small number of patients treated for malignant diseases with coincidental autoimmune disorders [41]. Autologous HSC transplantation has been performed for severe multiple sclerosis (MS) refractory to standard therapy with increasing frequency worldwide.

Accumulated information on clinical studies in Europe or the United States report relatively small numbers of patients, with less than 300 enrolled since 1997 worldwide. Existing data support the feasibility and promise of this procedure [42]. The recent extension of the HSC transplantation approach from rodents to humans for tolerance induction to alloantigens is highly encouraging. An understanding of the tolerization processes that apply to naive and memory T and B cells will ultimately lead to the development of less toxic, non myeloablative conditioning regimens. The development of such conditioning regimens will lead to new hope for patients in need of organ transplants and possibly for those with autoimmune diseases. The ultimate role for stem cell transplantation in the treatment of MS will be better defined by results of ongoing clinical trials, and by an improved understanding of disease pathogenesis, the genetic defects underlying different forms of autoimmune disease, and the mechanisms of tolerization of the memory T and B cells.

Immunomodulatory Drugs

There are currently six disease-modifying medications approved by the U.S. Food and Drug Administration (FDA) for use in relapsing forms of MS (including secondary-progressive MS). These include three interferon-β preparations [Avonex (Biogen Idec, Cambridge, Massachusetts, USA), Betaseron/Betaferon (Berlex, Montville, New Jersey, USA), and Rebif (Serono, Geneva, Switzerland)]; glatiramer acetate (GA, Copaxone; Teva, Petach Tikva, Israel); mitoxantrone (Novantrone; Serono, Geneva, Switzerland); and natalizumab (Tysabri; Biogen Idec) [5-10]. The interferon-βs (IFN-β) and GA serve as first-line agents, and have been in routine use for approximately a decade. The interferon-βs exert an anti-inflammatory effect by inhibiting cytokine production and limiting access of immune-cell infiltration into the central nervous system (CNS) [43-45]. GA induces changes in the phenotypic expression of T-helper cell populations and modifies central effects of inflammation [43-48]. These parenteral therapies are not reparative but preventive in action, and reduce MS relapses by one-third. All four drugs have demonstrated therapeutic efficacy in randomized controlled trials [5-8] and have an acceptable record of safety and tolerability. Mitoxantrone and nataluzimab are held in reserve as second-line MS therapies.

Both drugs have demonstrated efficacy in the treatment of MS [9, 10]; yet the potential for deleterious side effects has relegated their use to more aggressive forms of the disease [11, 49-53]. Unfortunately, none of the currently available disease-modifying drugs are approved for treating primary progressive MS—the type of MS that shows steady progression at onset. Several facts about immunomodulatory therapies are listed in Table 1.

Interferonβ-Based Therapies

IFN-β has been shown to modify the clinical relapse activity and disease progression in MS. Three genetically engineered drugs (Avonex, Betaseron and Rebif), introduced more than a decade ago, were the first members of a new generation of immunomodulators for MS [54]. IFN-β has proven to provide benefit in clinical trials in relapsing–remitting MS - those

Table 1. Immunomodulatory and Immunosuppressive Drugs Approved for Treatment of MS

Brand/generic name	Manufacturer/year of FDA approval	Indication/FDA-approved use	Frequency/Route of Delivery/Usual Dose
Avonex® / Interferon -1	Biogen Idec/1996	RR-MS[1]	Once a week/Intramuscular injection/30 g
Betaseron® / Interferon -1	Berlex Laboratories, Inc. / 1993	RR-MS and secondary-progressive MS	Every other day/subcutaneous injection/250 g
Copaxone® / glatiramer acetate	TEVA N euroscience, Inc. / 1996	RR-MS	Every day/subcutaneous injection/20 mg
Rebif® / / Interferon -1	Serono, Inc. / 2002	RR-MS	3 x week/subcutaneous injection/44 g
Tysabri® / Natalizumab	Biogen Idec and Elan Pharm., Inc. / 2006	RR-MS as monotherapy	Every four weeks/IV Infusion/300 mg
Novantrone®/ M itoxantrone	Serono, Inc. / 2000	Worsening RR/ secondary-progressive MS	Four times a year/IV Infusion/140 mg/3 y

[1] Relapsing-remitting MS.

taking the medication had a reduced risk of disability progression, experienced fewer exacerbations, and showed a reduction in number and size of active lesions in the brain (as shown on MRI) when compared with the group taking a placebo [5, 55, 56]. In a subsequent study of patients who had experienced a single demyelinating event in the optic nerve, spinal cord, or brainstem, and had lesions typical of MS on brain MRI, significantly delayed the time to a second exacerbation, and thus to a clinically definite diagnosis of MS. Moreover, IFN-β has also shown efficacy in patients with clinically isolated syndromes [2, 3], strengthening the case for early intervention. Finally, IFN-β appears to be moderately effective also in secondary progressive MS as long as superimposed relapses still reflect an ongoing inflammatory process [57-61].

The therapeutic clinical effects of IFN-β are mediated through a broad spectrum of its immunomodulatory activities. It is commonly accepted that IFN-β modulates antigen presentation by decreasing the expression of molecules, such as MHC class II on antigen presenting cells, and by downregulating co-stimulatory molecules. Moreover, IFN-β changes the expression pattern of cytokines released in the periphery, and it impacts the trafficking of inflammatory cells into the CNS by downregulating adhesion molecules, chemokines, and matrix metalloproteinases [62]. All these mechanisms would at least explain why IFN-β exhibits clinical efficacy in those clinical forms of MS that are associated with ongoing inflammation in the CNS. It has been proposed that IFN-β elicits neuroprotective functions both in vitro and in vivo [63, 64]. If one looks at brain atrophy measured by magnetic resonance imaging (MRI) as a surrogate marker for neuroprotection, treatment with IFN-β has revealed a significant impact in slowing down the progression of atrophy in some studies [65]. Similarly, evidence is available from clinical trials spanning up to 4 years that IFN-β influences clinical disease progression measured on the EDSS scale, indirectly pointing to a preservation or protection of neurons [56, 66]. It appears that any neuroprotection mediated by IFN-β reflects the anti-inflammatory effect of the drug executed within an early critical window of therapeutic opportunity. A better understanding of the sequential evolution of the MS lesion, its heterogeneity, and the development of clinical surrogate markers which would allow defining patients at higher risk and aiding in the identification of the underlying pathology, will lead to an improved treatment approach [67]. This would capitalize on currently approved and promising experimental drugs to effectively target the immunoinflammatory as well as neurodegenerative aspects of the disease process in MS.

Copaxone®: Laboratory and Clinical Findings

Copaxone® (GA) is widely used for the treatment of relapsing-remitting MS [68]. Data from several clinical trials have demonstrated its efficacy in reducing the relapse rate by about 30% and slowing progression of disability, as well as decreasing disease activity as monitored by MRI [8, 69-71]. In a recently published double-blind, randomized, multicentre study GA administered orally in relapsing-remitting multiple sclerosis (CORAL)] [72], the effect of two different oral doses of glatiramer acetate (50 mg or 5 mg once daily) were compared with placebo in 1644 patients with RRMS over 14 months. The study outcome was found not to differ between groups. Neither the cumulative number of confirmed relapses (primary end-point) nor several secondary and tertiary clinical and MRI parameters were different between the groups. Consequently, oral GA at the doses tested cannot be recommended for the treatment of RRMS. Several possible explanations may account for these disappointing results: the primary outcome power calculations may have been incorrect; the level of gut-associated immune responses induced by oral GA may be lower in patients than in experimental animal species [73]; or an inadequate dosage might have been chosen. The latter possibility is currently being addressed in a new trial testing a higher dose of oral GA in patients with RRMS.

A different study [49] evaluated the effect of GA given subcutaneously on accumulation of disability in primary progressive multiple sclerosis (PPMS). In this trial (named PROMiSe), a total of 943 patients with PPMS were randomly assigned to receive GA subcutaneously or placebo over 3 years. The trial failed to demonstrate a treatment effect of GA on PPMS. The study was halted after 2 years because findings at that time point indicated that treatment in the overall population was ineffective. One possible drawback of the study was that the observed annual progression rate on the Expanded Disability Status Scale was only 36%, which is markedly lower than the 50% annual progression rate estimate used for determining size and statistical power of the trial. The results from that study are in accordance with the unfortunate observation that modulation of the immune system is apparently ineffective in halting disease progression in PPMS [74].

GA is a random amino acid copolymer of alanine (A), lysine (K), glutamic acid (E), and tyrosine (Y) in a molar ratio of approximately 5:3:1.5:1 synthesized in solution using *N*-carboxyamino acid anhydrides [75]. Initially, this and other related four amino acid copolymers were used to define the genetic basis of immune responsiveness in genes now known as class II MHC locus [76, 77]. Later, GA was found to be effective both in the suppression of experimental allergic encephalomyelitis (EAE) in rodents and primates [78-80] and in the treatment of relapsing forms of MS [8, 69, 70]. Several mechanisms have been proposed to elucidate the inhibitory activity of GA. As a first step, its binding to class II MHC proteins on the surface of antigen-presenting cells (APC) has been demonstrated [81]. Importantly, GA bound extensively and in a promiscuous manner to mouse and human APC of various H-2 and HLA haplotypes. The specificity of the binding was confirmed by its inhibition with either the relevant anti-MHC class II antibodies or the unlabeled analogs. In addition, GA inhibited the binding of MS-associated immunodominant epitope p84-102 of the autoantigenic myelin basic protein (MBP) to the MHC class II molecules on human APC and even displaced the bound peptide [81]. In another study, GA was shown to inhibit binding of the two immunodominant epitopes of the major autoantigen in MS, the proteolipid protein (PLP) (p139-151 and p178-191), to the mouse I-A^s molecules, and to displace the

PLP peptides from the binding site [82]. Furthermore, the responses of T cell lines specific for these peptides were inhibited by GA in a dose-dependent manner. In vivo, GA affected the course of the chronic relapsing (CR)-EAE in (SJL/J x BALB/c)F1 mice, leading to almost complete resistance to the disease induction by either whole spinal cord homogenate or the above peptides [82]. GA exhibited a wide range of inhibition as it was shown to compete with several myelin antigens and their epitopes (MBP, PLP, MOG) for binding to class II MHC molecules and for activation of antigen-specific effector T cells [82, 83]. The capability of GA to bind to class II MHC molecules on the surface of APC without prior processing in vitro [84] was further substantiated by the observation on clustering of class II MHC in the presence of GA [85]. At the molecular level, GA was shown to bind to purified human HLA-DR1, DR2, and DR4 with high affinity in a temperature- and time -dependent manner, and was competitively inhibited by DR-restricted peptides, but not by peptide derivatives that bind with low affinity. Specifically, GA competed for binding of the immunodominant epitope of MBP, p85-99, to MS-associated HLA-DR2 (DRB1*1501) proteins and also inhibited the responses of DR2-restricted MBP-specific T cells. The formation of stable GA-DR complexes was demonstrated on SDS-PAGE [86]. These findings suggested that the effectiveness of GA in EAE and MS may be directly related to its binding to the groove of HLA-DR proteins.

In order to identify the amino acid sequence motifs of GA bound to the HLA-DR molecules, pool sequencing of GA-bound fragments eluted from MS-associated HLA-DR2 (DRB1*1501) and rheumatoid arthritis (RA)-associated HLA-DR1 (DRB1*0101) and HLA–DR4 (DRB1*0401) proteins has been performed [87]. In this elegant study, the protruding N-terminal ends of GA bound to recombinant empty HLA-DR1, -DR2, or -DR4 molecules, expressed in insect cells, were treated with aminopeptidase I, followed by elution, HPLC separation, and pool sequencing. In contrast to the untreated or unbound GA, which showed similar patterns of the amino acid composition and sequencing, the digested material exhibited distinct motifs at some positions within the binding site. Thus, there were increases in the levels of E at the first and second cycles, of K at the second and third cycles (corresponding to the P-1 position stabilizing the interactions of the bound peptide with the T Cell Receptor), and of Y (presumably at P1 of the bound peptide) at the third to fifth cycles, regardless of the HLA-DR molecule employed. No preference was seen at the following cycles that were mainly represented by A [87]. These pooled HLA-DR binding epitopes provided clues to the components of GA that are biologically active in suppressing MS and possibly RA.

Collectively, four major effects of GA in MS have been described: 1. Promiscuous binding to class II MHC molecules leading to competitive inhibition of other antigens [81, 86-88]. 2. Competition with MBP for binding to MBP-specific T cells (TCR antagonism, ref. 89). 3. Binding of GA/MHC complex on the surface of APC to T cells specific for several myelin antigens, in a manner similar to the altered peptide ligand (APL), leading to their anergy [90]. 4. Shift of Th1 to Th2 in GA-reactive regulatory T cells in vivo, resulting in suppressive bystander effect [91-94]. Major immunologic effects of GA reported up to date are listed in Table 2.

Table 2. Immunologic Effects of GA in MS

Effect	Reference
Direct and promiscuous binding to different HLA-DR alleles	[81, 86, 87]
Suppression of proliferation of MBP-specific T cells in vitro	[136]
Decreased proliferation of PBL to GA during treatment	[137-140]
Shift of GA-reactive T cells from Th1 to Th2 during treatment	[91]
Induction of cytokine production in MBP-specific T cells by GA	[91, 138]
TCR antagonism with MBP 86-100 epitope	[89]
Induction of anergy in MBP-specific T cell clones	[141]
Induction of immunomodulatory Th2 clones	[100-102]
Effects on APC: induction of differentiation/inhibition of reactivity	[142, 143]

GA-Related Copolymers and Their Mechanisms

Further investigation of the mechanisms involved in the activity of GA, as well as examination of additional synthetic copolymers has been carried out with the goal of developing improved therapeutic agents for MS. Novel peptides and copolymers have been designed on the basis of the binding motifs of GA and the autoantigenic peptides specific for MS and RA. In RA studies, peptides containing Y at P1 of the binding site were particularly effective as inhibitors of the binding of collagen type II p261-273 epitope (a candidate autoantigen in RA) to HLA-DR1 or –DR4 proteins. Moreover, several of the synthetic peptides were also potent inhibitors of the p261-273-reactive T cell clones [88]. In a different RA study, GA-related copolymers inhibited both the binding of p261-273 to RA-associated HLA-DR1 and –DR4 molecules and the response of DR1- and DR4-restricted p261-273-specific T cell clones [95]. In MS-related studies, peptides synthesized according to the binding motifs of GA and the immunodominant epitope of MBP p85-99, differentially inhibited binding of these antigens to disease-associated HLA-DR2 (DRB1*1501) molecules. In particular, two peptides with residue K at position P-1 inhibited effectively the binding of both MBP p85-99 and GA to the HLA-DR2 molecules, as well as decreased IL-2 production by the two MBP-specific HLA-DR2-restricted T-cell clones [96]. High-affinity modified synthetic peptide 15-mers inhibited even more strongly both the binding of MBP 85-99 to HLA-DR2 and IL-2 production by the two MBP 85-99-specific HLA-DR2-restricted T cells [93]. These peptides also suppressed EAE induced by MBP 85-99 in humanized mice, and PLP 139-151-induced EAE in SJL/J mice. Moreover, none of these peptide inhibitors cross-reacted with MBP 85-99- or PLP 139-151-specific T cells. In both cases, spleen and lymph node cultures stimulated with these peptides produced large amounts of Th2 cytokines (IL-4 and IL-10), and adoptive transfer of established T cell lines suppressed disease induction [97].

The effects and the mechanisms of GA-related copolymers composed of three or four amino acids have been examined in the EAE model. In the earlier study, the binding of copolymers to purified class II MHC molecules with differential affinities has been reported [98]. The three amino acid copolymer YAK bound to purified human HLA-DR1 or -DR4 molecules with affinity higher than YEA, EAK or YEK, whereas EAK was the better binder of HLA-DR2 molecules. On the other hand, YEA and YAK inhibited the binding of biotinylated GA to these molecules 10-fold more efficiently YEK. Finally, YEA, YAK and

EAK were cross-reactive with GA at the level of GA-specific T cell lines and clones of mouse or human origin [98]. In the subsequent study, 14-, 35-, and 50-mers of random sequences composed of four-amino acids at certain ratios have been synthesized as described above [99]. These copolymers were examined in three ways: (a) binding to "empty" HLA-DR2 (DRB1*1501) synthesized in a baculovirus system, (b) inhibition of the four MBP 85-99– or PLP 40-60–specific HLA-DR2–restricted T cell clones, as well as the two PLP 139-151–specific H-2^s–restricted T cell hybridomas, and finally (c) ability to suppress EAE induced by either PLP 139-151 or whole spinal cord homogenate (WSCH) in H-2^s mice. The following results were obtained: (a) In the binding experiment, VEAK and FEAK were less effective than GA (commercial batch) or YEAK (custom synthesized) in competing for binding of biotinylated MBP 86-100; (b) When tested as inhibitors of MBP 85-99– or PLP 40-60–induced stimulation of the four HLA-DR2–restricted T cell clones or hybridomas, VEAK was substantially less effective than GA or YEAK in inhibition of proliferation, while FEAK was equivalent to GA using two of these clones and slightly less effective in the other two cases. Using the two PLP 139-151–specific H-2^s–restricted T cell hybridomas, again FEAK was approximately equivalent to GA or YEAK, while VEAK was half as effective. In both the binding and the inhibition of T cell proliferation experiments, the 50-mers of all of the copolymers used were much more effective than the 35-mers or the 14-mers; (c) VEAK and GA were equally effective in partially reducing the severity of EAE induced by PLP 139-151 in H-2^s mice, while FEAK completely prevented the appearance of disease, except for a few mice who developed a transient +1 score (limp tail). In immunohistology, brain sections of control animals and VEAK-treated animals showed substantial demyelination, while animals treated with GA, YEAK, or FEAK were completely normal. WSCH was also used to induce the disease, in which case a milder disease was produced, perhaps more comparable to MS. The mild disease persisted in some animals treated with either GA or YEAK and in an even larger number of animals treated with VEAK. However, no disease was detected in any animals treated with FEAK [99].

Based on the above observations, additional copolymers have been designed as 50-mers. In this group, F was substituted for E because: (a) E seemed unnecessary. Moreover, the P1 pocket of DRB1*1501 includes β86Val, resulting in a small pocket that can accommodate F but for which Y is too large to be accommodated; (b) The residue occurring at P4 in MBP 85-99 is F, although Y would provide a better fit. To determine whether novel copolymers competed with the autoantigenic MS-associated epitope MBP 85-99 for binding to HLA-DR2, competitive binding assays were carried out with biotinylated MBP 86-100 and unlabeled random copolymers. All of the YFAK and FAK 50-mers were equally effective and equivalent to or better than any other copolymer or GA in binding to HLA-DR2. Moreover, YFAK and FAK were much more effective than GA in inhibition of MBP 85-99-specific HLA-DR2-restricted T cell clones. Most importantly, these novel copolymers YFAK and FAK were much more effective than GA in suppression of EAE induced in the susceptible SJL/J (H-2^s) mouse strain: none of the animals treated with YFAK developed significant disease. Furthermore, these copolymers have been shown to shift the immune responses of autoantigen-specific T cells from Th1 to Th2 phenotype, with IL-4 and IL-10 – characteristic cytokine profiles [100]. In the latter study, the enhanced efficacy of these copolymers in EAE induced in SJL/J mice with PLP 139-151 epitope was demonstrated by using three protocols: (i) simultaneous administration of autoantigen and copolymer (termed prevention), (ii) pretreatment with copolymers (vaccination), or (iii) administration of copolymers after disease onset (treatment). Strikingly, in the treatment protocol administration of soluble VWAK and YFAK after onset of disease led to stasis of its progression and suppression of histopathological evidence of EAE. In all of these protocols, the copolymers showed a pronounced suppressive effect on PLP 139–151-induced EAE in the order VWAK > YFAK >> GA.

The mechanisms by which these effects are achieved have been examined in several types of assays: binding of copolymers to I-A^s in competition with PLP 139-151 (blocking), cytokine production by T cells (T helper 2 polarization), and transfer of protection by $CD3^+$ splenocytes or, notably, by copolymer-specific T cell lines (induction of regulatory T cells). Importantly, these copolymers were shown to bind to I-A^s, the only class II MHC protein expressed in SJL/J mice and to cluster with and compete with PLP 139–151 for binding to I-A^s. Previously, aggregates (clusters) of I-A^s molecules after GA binding were detected on the surface of antigen-presenting cells from SJL/J mice [85]. YFAK and VWAK were more potent than GA in binding to mouse I-A^s molecules and in competing for PLP 139–151 binding. In addition to the competitive binding potential, the copolymers were also inhibitors of the expansion of PLP 139–151-specific T cells, both *in vitro* and *in vivo*, again in the order VWAK > YFAK > GA.

The generation of copolymer-specific regulatory T cells that secrete IL-4 and IL-10 and are independent of the immunizing autoantigen is very prominent among the multiple mechanisms that account for the observed suppressive effect of copolymers in EAE. Furthermore, copolymers shifted the T cell immune response from a classical Th1 phenotype toward a Th2 response (immune deviation). In SJL/J mice, re-stimulation of splenocytes from PLP 139–151-immunized animals with PLP 139–151 *in vitro* induced the production of IFN-γ but not IL-4 or IL-10. However, splenocytes from mice co-immunized with PLP 139–151 and copolymers when re-stimulated with their corresponding copolymers also produced IL-4 and IL-10 without much alteration in the production of IFN-γ. These cytokines may be produced by copolymer-specific T cells with a negligible contribution, if any, from PLP 139–151-reactive T cells. Third, copolymers may mediate their effects by inducing copolymer-specific T cells with the Th2 phenotype. The copolymers upon immunization of SJL/J mice induced a copolymer-specific T cell response, i.e., the copolymers are immunogenic. Moreover, adoptive transfer of copolymer-specific T cells reduced markedly the severity of EAE, suggesting that they produce Th2 cytokines without copolymer re-stimulation. Of note is that the copolymer-specific T cell lines are antigen nonspecific, i.e., they can be generated and they respond to copolymers in the absence of antigen. Thus, they may be useful in the treatment of other autoimmune diseases or in those where several autoantigens are involved, as is likely to be the case in MS.

However, whatever the mechanism, the first step must be binding to a class II MHC protein. The copolymers were optimized for binding to HLA-DR2 but they are likely to bind promiscuously to class II MHC proteins, including I-A^s, with varying affinities. A number of mechanisms, in addition to blocking and immune deviation, resulting from the generation of copolymer-specific T cells, such as TCR competition or induction of anergy, may be operative. Induction of hypo-responsive T cells (anergy) in MS patients after continuous administration of GA has been observed. The generation of copolymer-specific $CD4^+$ Th2 cell lines that secrete IL-4 and IL-10 and can adoptively transfer resistance to EAE appears very prominent among these mechanisms. Copolymers might also suppress disease through modulating CNS antigen-presenting cells i.e., microglia.

Different copolymers may have different mechanisms of suppression. VWAK appeared to be less able to generate T cell lines and also generates larger amounts of IL-4 and lower amounts of IFN-γ, yet it suppressed EAE somewhat more effectively. However, VWAK bound more tightly to I-A^s and thus might be a better blocking agent. YFAK was much more effective in stimulating copolymer-specific T cell lines and production of anti-inflammatory cytokines IL-4 and IL-10, and thus should be much more effective in disease reduction if immune deviation is the mechanism. Conversely, VWAK induced IL-4 and IL-10 production only relatively weakly and, like YFAK, also induced T cell anergy relatively poorly [100]. Thus, a combination of mechanisms may be involved in the reduction of severity of EAE. Altogether, these data suggested that random synthetic copolymers designed according to the binding motifs of the human immunodominant epitope MBP 85-99 and the binding pockets of HLA-DR2 might be more beneficial than GA in treatment of MS.

Mitoxantrone

Prior to its approval as a therapy in MS, Novantrone was used only to treat certain forms of cancer. Its activity involves suppression of the autoreactive T cells, B cells, and macrophages that are thought to lead the attack on the myelin sheath. The use of Novantrone for the treatment of MS has been evaluated in a series of European studies over a period of ten years. In a randomized, placebo-controlled, multi-center clinical trial involving patients with secondary-progressive or progressive-relapsing disease, participants received 12mg/m2 of Novantrone by short IV infusion once every three months for 24 months. Novantrone was found to delay the time to first treated relapse and time to disability progression. It also reduced the number of treated relapses and number of new lesions detected by magnetic resonance imaging. Based on findings from these studies, the FDA approved Novantrone in for reducing neurologic disability and/or the frequency of clinical relapses (attacks) in: (1) Patients with secondary progressive MS (disease that has changed from relapsing-remitting to progressive at a variable rate); (2) Progressive-relapsing MS (disease characterized by gradual increase in disability from onset with clear, acute relapses along the way); (3) Worsening relapsing-remitting MS (disease characterized by clinical attacks without complete remission, resulting in a step-wise worsening of disability). *Novantrone has not been approved for the treatment of primary-progressive MS* (characterized by progression from disease onset with no acute attacks or remissions).

In a different study, the clinical and MRI effects of mitoxantrone administered to 45 patients during the first five years of highly active relapsing-remitting MS were investigated [101]. Differences occurring between the end of treatment and follow-up were analyzed using parametric and non-parametric tests. One patient developed leukemia four months after the end of the treatment; no other serious adverse events occurred during treatment and the follow-up period. A clinically relevant reduction in the annualized relapse rate ($P<0.0001$ at end of treatment and $P<0.0001$ at follow-up) was found. At the end of treatment, 53% of patients experienced no increase in active lesions, while 73% showed no increase in the number of new lesions. At follow-up, 41 out of 45 (91%) patients showed a stable MRI pattern and were active-scan free. In summary, despite potential serious adverse events, e.g. induction of acute lymphoblastic leukemia [102], mitoxantrone might be considered an option in selected patients with very active early MS.

Natalizumab

Nataluzimab (Tysabri) is a humanized monoclonal antibody which targets a specific cell-surface adhesion molecule (very late antigen-4, VLA-4) on mononuclear cells and thereby prevents interaction with its endothelium-localized antigen vascular cell adhesion molecule 1 (VCAM-1). As a result, this agent dramatically reduces the trafficking of these cells into the CNS [10, 54, 103, 104]. Additional mechanisms, including impairment of T-cell reactivation and B-cell proliferation, are also conceivable [105-107]. In a randomized controlled trial, natalizumab markedly reduced clinical relapses and magnetic resonance imaging (MRI) lesions [10, 103], and heralded great promise as a new treatment option for MS patients. Unfortunately, the discovery of two cases of progressive multifocal leukoencephalopathy (PML) among MS patients treated with nataluzimab in combination with IFN-β [11, 51, 54] raised serious questions about its safety profile [103, 104], and the drug was temporarily withdrawn from clinical use [104]. Natalizumab has recently gained approval by the American FDA and European authorities (European Medicines Agency) as a monotherapy agent, but the potential long-term risks of this agent beyond 2 years is unknown [10, 11, 51, 54, 103].

Since a phase II proof-of-concept study suggested remarkable efficacy of the drug [108], two phase III trials of natalizumab in MS were initiated and recently reported [10, 54]. In the Natalizumab Safety and Efficacy in RR-MS (AFFIRM) trial [10], natalizumab was applied as a monotherapy (300 mg intravenous or placebo every 28 days for up to 28 months) in 942 MS patients who had not received any immunotherapy during the preceding 6 months. Of patients in the treatment arm 96% were devoid of new gadolinium-enhancing lesions, as compared with 68% in the placebo group. Relapse frequency was reduced by approximately two-thirds over years 1 and 2, and natalizumab also significantly delayed disease progression. The Safety and Efficacy of Natalizumab in Combination with IFN-β1α in Patients with Relapsing Remitting Multiple Sclerosis (SENTINEL) study [54] compared the combination of natalizumab with IFN-β1α intramuscularly once weekly versus IFN-β1α alone. Patients receiving IFN-β1α were randomly assigned to receive either natalizumab 300 mg (n = 589) or placebo (n = 582) every 28 days. In those receiving combination therapy relapse rate reduced by 54% compared with those on IFN-β1α monotherapy; they also had significantly fewer MRI lesions. Adverse events in both studies included anaphylactoid reactions, rash, arthralgia and headache.

Based on the positive interim analyses of both phase III trials, natalizumab was approved by the FDA for the treatment of 'relapsing forms of multiple sclerosis' in November 2004. In February 2005, however, the substance was withdrawn from the market because two patients receiving natalizumab along with IFN-β1α developed progressive multifocal leucoencephalopathy (PML) [11, 51]. Consequently, an extensive re-examination of all patients who had received natalizumab in clinical trials in the settings of RRMS and Crohn's disease was performed, examining various safety aspects (clinical, laboratory and MRI) [109]. No additional cases of PML were identified in more than 3000 patients exposed to the drug over a period of 18 months on average. Based on these findings, in June 2006 the US FDA approved an application to resume marketing of natalizumab as monotherapy in patients with 'relapsing forms of multiple sclerosis who have not responded adequately to, or cannot tolerate other treatments'. To minimize the risk for further serious adverse events, a special restricted distribution program and the risk management plan Tysabri Outreach Unified Commitment to Health (TOUCH) were implemented in the USA [110]. In Europe, natalizumab has been approved by the European Medicines Agency as monotherapy for patients with high disease activity despite sufficient treatment with IFN-β as well as for patients with initially high disease activity.

The advent of natalizumab for the treatment of MS opens a new era of immune-specific therapy. The current situation is unique, however, because the high efficacy of this mAb is associated with an uncertain safety profile, especially with long-term administration. Natalizumab interferes with a critical step in MS disease pathogenesis, namely entry of encephalitogenic T cells to the CNS compartment. Because of its mechanism of action, the substance may impede immune surveillance of the CNS. It is unknown, however, whether a virus reactivation (or de-novo infection) was caused by general immunosuppression, or by a more specific effect related to the particular mode of action of this drug (mobilization of cells containing the virus from the BM) [111, 112]. Clearly, it is important that much more is learned about virus infections and attendant immunological changes so that we may better assess the benefit–risk ratio [113] and design clinical strategies [114].

Combinational Therapy

The pathophysiology of MS is multifaceted, and combining different drugs with complementary mechanisms of action may be needed to exert maximal clinical benefit in patients who do not respond to conventional monotherapies. The principal clinical rationale for using drug combinations is to obtain additive or even synergistic therapeutic effects [115]. There are two pharmacological rationales for using a combination of two or more drugs: Class 1 combination therapies include two (or more) drugs that are considered independent of each other and target different aspects of the injurious mechanisms underlying the disease [116]. In the case of MS, for example, one drug might target cell trafficking into the CNS, whereas another drug might affect cell activation. Class 2 drug combinations include two or more pharmacological agents that have distinct molecular targets within a single cell type, or a single response pathway in that cell type [116].

The biological effects of the vast majority of pharmacological agents are mediated by interactions of their specific receptors. These may include classical drug receptors for hormones and neurotransmitters, or non-classical drug receptors that obey the laws of drug–receptor interactions. The formation of drug–receptor complexes defines the cellular and clinical effects of pharmacotherapy. Increased activation of a drug–receptor complex occurs through the combination of agonistic pharmacological agents, whereas antagonist drugs do not alter the activation status of drug–receptor complexes. Antagonistic substances can still result in clinically important effects, because by binding to a receptor site they can prevent agonists from increasing drug–receptor-complex activation. In a third scenario, a pharmacological agent binds and activates a receptor, but elicits a suboptimal biological response. These drugs are called partial agonists. Notably, partial agonists with low efficacy often behave as antagonists. Given that the biological net result of combination therapy with different agents may be difficult to predict it is critical to eliminate potential antagonism in preclinical studies.

Efforts are ongoing to establish a role for combination therapies in MS, yet data are currently lacking. Most trials to date have been uncontrolled observational studies [44, 45]. The hypothesis that combining agents with complementary or synergistic effects may improve therapeutic efficacy needs to be tested in randomized control trials if combination treatment strategies are to have any resounding impact in the management of MS patients. Most ongoing studies include IFN-β or GA in combination with other potent immunosuppressant agents (including mitoxantrone, cyclophosphamide, methotrexate, or aziathoprine [43]), or with an agent with a distinctly different mechanism of action, including monoclonal antibodies [49].

The only large-scale controlled trial of combination therapy in MS was the SENTINEL study, which randomized 1200 MS patients on IFN-β1α (Avonex) with persistent disease activity to receive IFN-β1α alone or in combination with natalizumab (300 mg monthly, administered intravenously) for 2 years [54]. Patients who received the combination therapy demonstrated fewer relapses and improved MRI markers of disease activity compared with patients treated with IFN-β1α alone [54]. Unfortunately, two of the MS patients treated with the combination therapy developed PML [43, 44, 49, 54]. The outcome of this study heightened our awareness regarding the perils of combining drugs, particularly in standard monotherapy doses, with the potential to exert robust synergistic immunosuppressive effects.

Given its distinct mechanisms of action, GA may represent the ideal candidate to partner with other agents to achieve complementary and potentially synergistic therapeutic effects. Boggild and colleagues [43, 117] used mitoxantrone as an induction therapy followed by maintenance therapy with GA in a nonrandomized, uncontrolled observational case series, and observed a 90% reduction in relapse rate among patients. The potential applications of mitoxantrone and GA are currently being explored in two combination therapy trials: the first is the NC100 study, which will compare the effects of mitoxantrone induction followed by a GA regimen with treatment with GA alone in 40 patients with relapsing MS. The primary goal of this study is to generate safety and MRI data [43]. The second study is the United Kingdom Early Mitoxantrone Copaxone Trial, which will randomize 60–100 patients to receive either combination treatment (mitoxantrone and GA) or IFN-β1α (Rebif) as monotherapy for a period of 3 years [43]. The National Institutes of Health is currently funding the first large-scale (Class I) multicenter clinical trial testing the combined use of IFN-β1α (Avonex) and GA (Copaxone) to treat relapsing MS [43-45, 49]. The combination therapy will be compared with the use of either agent alone for a period of 3 years. A previous multicenter, open-label trial demonstrated that the combination of GA and IFN-β1α (Avonex) was safe in MS patients [44, 118].

Previous pilot studies have used IFN-β in combination with azathioprine, corticosteroids, cyclophosphamide and mitoxantrone [44, 45, 119], and larger-scale trials are underway to better elucidate the role of IFN-β in combination therapy protocols. An open-label study combined methotrexate and IFN-β1α (Avonex), and demonstrated reduced relapse rates and improved MRI measures of disease activity in patients treated with methotrexate as an additive therapy [43, 120]. A multicenter, placebo-controlled study (the Avonex Combination Trial) is now underway to determine both the safety and efficacy of combining IFN-β1α (Avonex) with intravenous methylprednisolone, oral methotrexate or both in MS patients [44, 45].

Italian investigators have initiated three multicenter controlled trials using IFN-β in combination therapies. The first is a single-blind study designed to evaluate the safety and efficacy of induction therapy with monthly methotrexate followed by IFN-β1α (Rebif). This study will select MS patients early in their disease course with more deleterious clinical prognostic factors or MRI markers of disease activity. Patients will be treated either with IFN-β 1α monotherapy or a 6-month induction of mitoxantrone followed by IFN-β1α at the same dosage and frequency. The primary endpoints of the study are to determine the proportion of relapse-free patients after 2 years, and the number of patients with confirmed clinical worsening after 4 years [49]. The second single-blind study will compare the effects of IFN-β combined with cyclophosphamide therapy to IFN-β monotherapy in 225 patients who are deemed to be 'partial' or 'nonresponders' to IFN-β therapy alone [49]. The third study is designed to compare the combination therapy of IFN-β and azathioprine with IFN-β monotherapy in 85 patients with secondary progressive MS. Patients will be followed to compare clinical and MRI outcome measures for 3 years [49].

Future Perspectives: Candidate Therapies

Numerous combination therapies are currently being evaluated in controlled clinical settings. These are available for review on the National Multiple Sclerosis Society website (www.nationalmssociety. org/Clinical%20Trials.asp). All combinations include at least one approved agent, and one experimental drug or another approved therapeutic. Examples include treatment of MS with GA (Copaxone) and albuterol, IFN-β1α (Avonex) plus mycophenolate mofetil (CellCept), immunotherapy with BHT-3009 alone or combined with atorvastatin (Lipitor), and minocycline plus GA (Copaxone). Other candidate agents for combination therapies include vitamin B_{12}, low-fat diet with omega-3 supplements, antioxidant agents, hormonal therapies and folic acid [45, 49].

Ongoing Clinical Trials

A number of novel immunomodulators are currently being examined in clinical trials for efficacy in MS, most of them representing small molecules that specifically target a critical checkpoint in the immunopathogenic cascade of MS. Published data are limited at present, however, they fuel hopes that these drugs may broaden our therapeutic armamentarium. A pipeline of 17 drugs in various phases of development is currently being investigated in clinical trials for MS. These include interferons and other immune system modulators, as well as a few drugs aimed at symptomatic relief, which are summarized in Table 3.

Recent advances in molecular biology and genetics have paid dividends for research in MS therapeutics. By targeting specific pathways thought to be involved in myelin destruction, one or more of these agents may ultimately prove to be a "silver bullet" reducing or preventing relapses while maintaining a reasonably good safety and tolerability profile. For the agents in earlier phases of development, only time will tell to what extent these disease-modifying drugs may accomplish these goals.

Table 3. Candidate Drugs Tested in Ongoing Clinical Trials

Candidate Drug	Clinical trial/Indication	Frequency/Dose/Route of Delivery	Outcome/In progress	Reference (If applicable)
ZK81 1752 (CC chemokine receptor 1antagonist BX-471)	Multicenter, randomized, double-blind, phase II/ RRMS	three times daily/600 mg/oral/ placebo90 patients/16weeks efficacy on several MRI para meters of disease activity	was well tolerated but failed todemonstratesignificant	121-125
FTY 720 (fingolimod)	Multicenter, double-blind, Placebo-controlled, phase II/ RRM S	1.25 mg/day or 5 mg/day/oral/ 281 patients/6 months	MRI lesion s were significantly Improved, the relapse ratewas decreasedby 55%	126-134
Sativex (GW-1000, Tetranabinex) by GW Pharmaceuticals	Placebo-controlled, phase III/ RRMS	sublingual spray/ 350 patients/52 weeks/	safe and effective, with improvement in spasticity compared with placebo	
My linax (cladribine) By IVA X/Serono	A two-year, double-blind, placebo-controlled phase III / RRMS	oral/> 1,200 patients	ongoing/relapses, progression of disability, serial MRI sca ns	
MBP8298 (synthetic MBP peptide) By BioMS Medical	Phase II/III/RR MS	high dose/intravenously	statistically significant clinical benefit in Phase II	
Rituximab By Genentech	Phase II/III/PPMS	intravenously	temporarily suppressed the activation of B cells in cerebrospinal fluid	135
ATL110 2 (antisense inhibitor of VLA-4) by Antisense Therapeutics	Double-blind, dose-escalation/ placebo-controlledPhase I	6mg/kg/week/ 54 healthyvolunteers	well tolerated andwould be an appropriate dosefor Phase II development	
	Multicenter, double-blinded/ Phase IIa/RRMS	400 mg/week/twice weekly/ subcu taneous/60 patients/8 weeks	monthly MRI	
Alferon N(IFN -n3) by Hemispherx Biopharma	Phase IIa/RRMS	subcutaneous/38 untreated/ 31 treatedpatients/36 months	MRI lesion s decreased EDS S decreased from 4.8 to 3.4	
Fampridine SR by Acorda Therapeutics	Phase II/RR MS	oral, sustained-release tablet formulation of 4-aminopyridine	faster walking andimproved leg strength	
Laquinimod by Active Biotech/Teva	Phase II /RRMS	oral/24 weeks	28% to 44% reduction in new brain MRI lesio ns	
ABT-874 (anti-I L-12) By Abbott Laboratories	Randomized/ Phase I/RRMS	48 weeks	ongoing/MRI lesio ns	
Campath-1H (anti-CD5 2) By Genzyme	Secondary-progressive MS RR MS	intravenously/27 patients low/high dose/intravenously/ 180 patients	no new lesions for 18 months 1/3 of patients developed Graves disease	
NeuroVax (I R208) by Immune Response Corp.	multicenter, three-arm, randomized Phase II/RRMS	60 patients/24 weeks	was well tolerated with no serious adverse effects	
Pirfenidone (TNF- inh) By InterMune	open-label/Phase II/ chronic progressive MS	20 patients/two-year study	Improvement and stabilization at 3 months, was sustained atsix, 1 2 and 24 months	
Zenapax(daclizumab) By ProteinDesign Labs	Phase II recruiting	Intravenously	recruitingpatients	

Concluding Remarks

More-effective therapies are needed to treat MS patients. Until our understanding of MS pathogenesis advances, and novel molecular targets are identified, combinations of approved and experimental agents may provide a viable treatment strategy. Combination therapies have been established as the standard of care in other autoimmune diseases. There are now numerous rationales for the use of combination therapy in MS, and the pharmacologic principles for evaluating and understanding their actions are available. By applying these principles, the development of novel combinations that are safe and more efficacious than existing monotherapies appears to be an achievable goal. There is currently insufficient evidence regarding the safety and efficacy of combination therapies in MS. Therefore, the evaluation of specific combination therapies in the setting of well-designed clinical trials should be a priority for pharmacological companies and academia.

It would be premature to launch clinical trials to use stem cells to treat neurological disorders. However, steady progress supports the hope that stem-cell-based therapies to restore and preserve function in the brain and spinal cord can be developed. For each disease, it is now possible to develop a road map that defines the necessary scientific and clinical advances required for stem cells to reach the clinic [144]. Before we apply stem-cell therapies to patients, we must be able to control the proliferation and differentiation of stem cells into specific cellular phenotypes and to prevent tumour formation. Furthermore, the efficacy of stem cells and their mechanisms of action should be demonstrated in animal models with pathology and manifestations resembling the human disease. Even so, it may be difficult to translate data obtained in animals to humans because of species differences in the degree of neuronal plasticity and an incomplete knowledge of disease mechanisms. We must understand how to influence the pathological tissue environment, including inflammatory and immune reactions, to allow efficient repair. Finally, we must remember that however exciting the neurobiological mechanisms might be, the clinical usefulness of stem cells will be determined by their ability to provide patients with neurological disorders with safe, long-lasting and substantial improvements in quality of life.

References

[1] Jacobs, LD; Beck, RW; Simon, JH; et al. Intramuscular interferon beta-1α therapy initiated during a first demyelinating event in multiple sclerosis. CHAMPS Study Group. *N. Engl. J. Med.*, 2000, 343, 898–904.

[2] Comi, G; Filippi, M; Barkhof, F; et al. Effect of early interferon treatment on conversion to definite multiple sclerosis: a randomized study. *Lancet,* 2001, 357, 1576–1582.

[3] Kappos, L; Polman, CH; Freedman, MS; et al. Treatment with interferon beta-1β delays conversion to clinically definite and McDonald MS in patients with clinically isolated syndromes. *Neurology*, 2006, 67, 1242–1249.

[4] Frohman, EM; Havrdova, E; Lublin F, et al. Most patients with multiple sclerosis or a clinically isolated syndrome should be treated at the time of diagnosis. *Arch. Neurol.*, 2006, 63, 614–619.

[5] Jacobs, LD; Cookfair, DL; Rudick, RA; et al. Intramuscular interferon beta-1a for disease progression in relapsing multiple sclerosis: the Multiple Sclerosis Collaborative Research Group (MSCRG). *Ann. Neurol.*, 1996, 39, 285–294.

[6] IFN[beta] Multiple Sclerosis Study Group. Interferon beta-1β is effective in relapsing remitting multiple sclerosis. I. Clinical results of a multicenter, randomized, double-blind, placebo-controlled trial. *Neurology*, 1993, 43, 655–661.

[7] PRISMS (Prevention of Relapses and Disability by Interferon beta 1a Subcutaneously in Multiple Sclerosis) Study Group. Randomized double-blind placebo-controlled study

of interferon beta 1a in relapsing/remitting multiple sclerosis. *Lancet*, 1998, 352, 1498–1504.

[8] Johnson, KP; Brooks, BR; Cohen, JA; et al. Copolymer 1 reduces relapse rate and improves disability in relapsing-remitting multiple sclerosis: results of a phase III multicenter, double-blind placebo controlled trial. The Copolymer Multiple Sclerosis Study Group. *Neurology*, 1995, 45, 1268–1276.

[9] Hartung, HP; Gonsette, R; Kongi, N; et al. Mitoxantrone in progressive multiple sclerosis: a placebo-controlled, double-blind, randomized, multicenter trial. *Lancet*, 2002, 360, 2018–2025.

[10] Polman, CH; O'Connor, PW; Havrdova, E; et al. A randomized, placebo-controlled trial of natalizumab for relapsing multiple sclerosis. *N. Engl. J. Med.*, 2006, 354, 899–910.

[11] Langer-Gould, A; Atlas, SW; Green, AJ; et al. Progressive multifocal leukoencephalopathy in a patient treated with natalizumab. *N. Engl. J. Med.*, 2005, 353, 375–381.

[12] Lubetzki, C., Williams, A; Stankoff, B. Promoting repair in multiple sclerosis: problems and prospects. *Curr. Opin. Neurol.*, 2005, 18, 237–244.

[13] Trapp, B; Ransohof, R; Rudick, R. Axonal pathology in multiple sclerosis: relationship to neurologic disability, *Curr. Opin. Neurol.* 1999, 12, 295–302.

[14] Lovas, G; Szilagyi, N; Majtenyi, K; *et al.*, Axonal changes in chronic demyelinated cervical spinal cord plaques. Brain, 2000, 123, 308–317.

[15] Grigoriadis, N; Ben-Hur, T; Karussis, D; *et al.*, Axonal damage in multiple sclerosis: a complex issue in a complex disease. Clin. Neurol. Neurosurg., 2004, 106, 211–217.

[16] Steinman, L. Multiple sclerosis: a two-stage disease. Nat. Immunol., 2001, 2, 762–764.

[17] Owens, T. The enigma of multiple sclerosis: inflammation and neurodegeneration cause heterogeneous dysfunction and damage. Curr. Opin. Neurol., 2003, 16, 259–265.

[18] Felts, P; Woolston, A; Fernando, H; *et al.*, Inflammation and primary demyelination induced by the intraspinal injection of lipopolysaccharide. *Brain,* 2005, 128, 1649–1666.

[19] Bitsch, A; Schuchardt, J; Bunkowski, S; *et al.*, Acute axonal injury in multiple sclerosis. Correlation with demyelination and inflammation. *Brain,* 2000, 123, 1174–1183.

[20] Bjartmar, C; Trapp, B. Axonal and neuronal degeneration in multiple sclerosis: mechanisms and functional consequences, Curr. Opin. Neurol., 2001, 14, 271–278.

[21] Buntinx, M; Stinissen, P; Steels, P; *et al.*, Immune-mediated oligodendrocyte injury in multiple sclerosis: molecular mechanisms and therapeutic interventions. *Crit. Rev. Immunol.*, 2002, 22, 391–424.

[22] Hohlfeld, R; Kerschensteiner, M; Stadelmann, C; *et al.*, The neuroprotective effect of inflammation: implications for the therapy of multiple sclerosis. *J. Neuroimmunol.*, 2000, 107, 161–166.

[23] Villoslada, P; Genain, G. Role of nerve growth factor and other trophic factors in brain inflammation. *Prog. Brain. Res.*, 2004, 146, 403–414.

[24] Einstein, O; Karussis, D; Grigoriadis, N; *et al.* Intraventricular transplantation of neural precursor cell spheres attenuates acute experimental allergic encephalomyelitis. *Mol. Cell. Neurosci.*, 2003, 24, 1074–1082.

[25] Pluchino, S; Quattrini, A; Brambilla, E; *et al.* Injection of adult neurospheres induces recovery in a chronic model of multiple sclerosis. *Nature,* 2003, 422, 688–694.

[26] Ben-Hur, T; Einstein, O; Mizrachi-Kol, R; *et al.* Transplanted multipotential neural precursor cells migrate into the inflamed white matter in response to experimental autoimmune encephalomyelitis. *Glia,* 2003, 41, 73–80.

[27] Prockop, D. Marrow stromal cells as stem cells for nonhematopoietic tissues. *Science,* 1997, 276, 71–74.

[28] Bonnet, D. Biology of human bone marrow stem cells. Clin. Exp. Med., 2003, 3, 140–149.

[29] McKay, RG. Stem cells in the central nervous system. *Science,* 1997, 276, 66–71.

[30] Gottlieb, DI. Large scale sources of neural stem cells. *Annu. Rev. Neurosci.,* 2002, 25, 381–407.

[31] Kim, SU. Genetically engineered human neural stem cells for brain repair in neurological diseases. Brain and Development, 2007, 29, 193-201.

[32] Windrem, MS; *et al.* Fetal and adult human oligodendrocyte progenitor cell isolates myelinate the congenitally dysmyelinated brain. *Nature Med.,* 2004, 10, 93–97.

[33] Back, SA; *et al.* Hyaluronan accumulates in demyelinated lesions and inhibits oligodendrocyte progenitor maturation. *Nature Med.,* 2005, 11, 966–972.

[34] Nistor, GI; Totoiu, MO; Haque, N; Carpenter, MK; Keirstead, HS. Human embryonic stem cells differentiate into oligodendrocytes in high purity and myelinate after spinal cord transplantation. *Glia,* 2005, 49, 385–396.

[35] Pluchino, S; *et al.* Neurosphere-derived multipotent precursors promote neuroprotection by an immunomodulatory mechanism. *Nature,* 2005, 436, 266–271.

[36] Karussis, D; Grigoriadis, S; Polyzoidou, E; Grigoriadis, N; Slavin, S; Abramsky, O. Neuroprotection in multiple sclerosis. Clin. Neurol. Neurosurg., 2006, 108, 250-254.

[37] Zhang, J; Li, Y; Chen, J; *et al.* Human bone marrow stromal cell treatment improves neurological functional recovery in EAE mice. *Exp. Neurol.* 2005, 195,16–26.

[38] Zappia, E; Casazza, S; Pedemonte, E; *et al.* Mesenchymal stem cells ameliorate experimental autoimmune encephalomyelitis inducing T cell anergy. *Blood,* 2005, 106, 1755–1761.

[39] Kanwar, J; Kanwar, R; Krissansen, G. Simultaneous neuroprotection and blockade of inflammation reverses autoimmune encephalomyelitis. *Brain,* 2004, 127, 1313–1331.

[40] Lindvall, O; Kokaia, Z. Stem cells for the treatment of neurological disorders. *Nature,* 2006, 441, 1094-1096.

[41] Sykes, M; Nicolic, B. Treatment of severe autoimmune disease by stem-cell transplantation. Nature, 2005, 435, 620-627.

[42] Loh, YS; Hwang, WY; Ratnagopal, P. Autologous haematopoietic stem cell transplantation for the treatment of multiple sclerosis. *Ann. Acad. Med. Singapore,* 2007, 36, 421-426.

[43] Boggild, M. Rationale and experience with combination therapies in multiple sclerosis. *J. Neurol.*, 2006, 253, VI/45–VI/51.

[44] Tullman, MJ; Lublin, FD. Combination therapy in multiple sclerosis. *Curr. Neurol. Neurosci. Rep.*, 2005, 5, 245–248.

[45] Weinstock-Guttman, B; Bakshi, R. Combination therapy for multiple sclerosis. *CNS Drugs*, 2004, 18, 777–792.

[46] Kieseier, BC; Wiendl, H; Hemmer, B; Hartung, HP. Treatment and treatment trials in multiple sclerosis. *Curr. Opin. Neurol.*, 2007, 20, 3, 286-293.

[47] Cohen, JA; Rovaris, M; Goodman, AD; Ladkani, D; Wynn, D; Filippi, M; 9006 Study Group. Randomized, double-blind, dose-comparison study of glatiramer acetate in relapsing-remitting MS. *Neurology*, 2007, 68, 939-944.
[48] Wolinsky, JS; Narayana, PA; O'Connor, P; Coyle, PK; Ford, C; Johnson, K; Miller, A; Pardo, L; Kadosh, S; Ladkani, D; PROMiSe Trial Study Group. Glatiramer acetate in primary progressive multiple sclerosis: results of a multinational, multicenter, double-blind, placebo-controlled trial. *Ann. Neurol.*, 2007, 61, 1, 14-24.
[49] Martinelli, V. Combination therapy. *Neurol. Sci.*, 2006, 27, S350–S354.
[50] Kleinschmidt-Demasters, BK; Tyler, KL. Progressive multifocal leukoencephalopathy complicating treatment with natalizumab and interferon beta-1α for multiple sclerosis. *N. Engl. J. Med.*, 2005, 353, 369–374.
[51] Van Assche, G; Van Ranst, M; Sciot, R; *et al.* Progressive multifocal leukoencephalopathy after natalizumab therapy for Crohn's disease. *N. Engl. J. Med.*, 2005, 353, 362–368.
[52] Rudick, RA; Stuart, WH; Calabresi, PA; *et al.* Natalizumab plus interferon beta-1α for relapsing multiple sclerosis. *N. Engl. J. Med.*, 2006, 354, 911–923.
[53] Hemme, B; Frohman, EM; Hartung, HP; *et al.* Central nervous system infections – a potential complication of systemic immunotherapy. *Curr. Opin. Neurol.*, 2006, 19, 271-276.
[54] Kieseier, BC; Hartung, HP. Current disease-modifying therapies in multiple sclerosis. *Semin. Neurol.,* 2003, 23, 133–146.
[55] PRISMS Study Group. Randomised double-blind placebo-controlled study of interferon beta-1a in relapsing/remitting multiple sclerosis. *Lancet,* 1998, **352,** 1498–1504.
[56] PRISMS Study Group, PRISMS-4: long-term efficacy of interferon-beta-1a in relapsing MS. *Neurology,* 2001, 56, 1628–1636.
[57] Cohen, JA; Cutter, GR; Fischer, JS; Goodman, AD; Heidenreich, FR; Kooijmans, MF; *et al.* Benefit of interferon beta-1a on MSFC progression in secondary progressive MS. *Neurology,* 2002, 59, 679–687.
[58] Anonymous, European Study Group on interferon beta-1β in secondary progressive multiple sclerosis. Placebo-controlled multicenter randomised trial of interferon beta-1β in treatment of secondary progressive multiple sclerosis. *Lancet,* 1998, 352, 1491–1497.
[59] Kappos, L; Weinshenker, B; Pozzilli, C; Thompson, AJ; Dahlke, F; Beckmann, K; *et al.* Interferon beta-1β in secondary progressive MS: a combined analysis of the two trials. *Neurology,* 2004, 63, 1779–1787.
[60] Panitch, H; Miller, A; Paty, D; Weinshenker, B; North American Study Group on interferon beta-1b in secondary progressive MS. Interferon beta-1b in secondary progressive MS: results from a 3-year controlled study. *Neurology,* 2004, 63, 1788–1795.
[61] SPECTRIMS Study Group. Randomized controlled trial of interferon-beta-1a in secondary progressive MS: clinical results. *Neurology,* 2001, 56, 1496–1504.
[62] Yong, VW. Differential mechanisms of action of interferon-beta and glatiramer acetate in MS. *Neurology,* 2002, 59, 802–808.
[63] Biernacki, K; Antel, JP; Blain, M; Narayanan, S; Arnold, DL; Prat, A. Interferon beta promotes nerve growth factor secretion early in the course of multiple sclerosis. *Arch. Neurol.,* 2005, 62, 119–124.

[64] Sättler, MB; Demer, I; Williams, SK; Maier, K; Merkler, D; Gadjanski, I; *et al.* Effects of interferon-beta-1a on neuronal survival under autoimmune inflammatory conditions. *Exp. Neurol.,* 2006, 201, 172–181.
[65] Rudick, R; Fisher, E; Lee, J; Simon, J; Jacobs, LD. Use of the brain parenchymal fraction to measure whole brain atrophy in relapsing–remitting MS. *Neurology,* 1999, 53, 1698–1704.
[66] Rudick, RA; Goodkin, DE; Jacobs, LD; Cookfair, DL; Herndon, RM; Richert, JR; *et al.* Impact of interferon beta-1a on neurologic disability in relapsing multiple sclerosis. The Multiple Sclerosis Collaborative Research Group (MSCRG). *Neurology,* 1997, 49, 358–363.
[67] Hohlfeld, R; Wekerle, H. Autoimmune concepts of multiple sclerosis as a basis for selective immunotherapy: from pipe dreams to (therapeutic) pipelines. *Proc. Natl. Acad. Sci. USA.,* 2004, 101, S14599–S14606.
[68] Perumal, J; Filippi, M; Ford, C; Johnson, K; Lisak, R; Metz, L; Tselis, A; Tullman, M; Khan, O. Glatiramer acetate therapy for multiple sclerosis: a review. *Expert Opin. Drug. Metab. Toxicol.,* 2006, 2, 1019-1029.
[69] Bornstein, MB; Miller, A; Slagle, S; et al. A pilot trial of COP 1 in exacerbating-remitting multiple sclerosis. *N. Engl. J. Med.*, 1987, 317, 408–414.
[70] Johnson, KP; Brooks, BR; Cohen, JA; et al. Extended use of glatiramer acetate (Copaxone) is well tolerated and maintains its clinical effect on multiple sclerosis relapse rate and degree of disability. The Copolymer 1 Multiple Sclerosis Study Group. *Neurology,* 1998, 50, 701–708.
[71] Comi, G; Filippi, M. The effect of glatiramer acetate (Copaxone) on disease activity as measured by cerebral MRI in patients with relapsing-remitting multiple sclerosis (RRMS): A multi-center, randomized, double blind, placebo-controlled study extended by open-label treatment. *Neurology,* 1999, 56 (suppl 2), 289.
[72] Filippi, M; Wolinsky, JS; Comi, G. Effects of oral glatiramer acetate on clinical and MRI-monitored disease activity in patients with relapsing multiple sclerosis: a multicentre, double-blind, randomised, placebo-controlled study. *Lancet Neurol.*, 2006, 5, 213–220.
[73] Hafler, DA; Weiner, HL. Immunologic mechanisms and therapy in multiple sclerosis. *Immunol. Rev.*, 1995, 144, 75–107.
[74] Leary, SM; Thompson, AJ. Primary progressive multiple sclerosis: current and future treatment options. *CNS Drugs*, 2005, 19, 369–376.
[75] Teitelbaum, D; Meshorer, A; Hirshfeld, T; Arnon, R; Sela, M. Suppression of experimental allergic encephalomyelitis by a synthetic polypeptide. *Eur. J. Immunol.*, 1971, 1, 242-248.
[76] McDevitt, HO; Sela, M. Genetic control of the antibody response. I. Demonstration of determinant-specific differences in response to synthetic polypeptide antigens in two strains of inbred mice. *J. Exp. Med.*, 1965, 122, 517-532.
[77] McDevitt, HO; Sela, M. Genetic control of the antibody response. II. Further analysis of the specificity of determinant-specific control, and genetic analysis of the response to (H,G)-A—L in CBA and C57 mice. *J. Exp. Med.*, 1967, 126, 969-978.
[78] Teitelbaum, D; Webb, C; Meshorer, A; Arnon, R; Sela, M. Suppression by several polypeptides of experimental allergic encephalomyelitis induced in guinea pigs and

rabbits with bovine and human basic encephalitogen. *Eur. J. Immunol.*, 1973, 3, 273-279.

[79] Teitelbaum, D; *et al.* Suppression of experimental allergic encephalomyelitis in rhesus monkeys by a synthetic basic copolymer. *Clin. Immunol. Immunopathol.*, 1974, 3, 256-262.

[80] Keith, AB; Arnon, R; Teitelbaum, D; Caspary, EA, Wisniewski HM. The effect of Cop 1, a synthetic polypeptide, on chronic relapsing experimental allergic encephalomyelitis in guinea pigs. *J. Neurol. Sci.*, 1979, 42, 267–274.

[81] Fridkis-Hareli, M; Teitelbaum, D; Gurevich, E; Pecht, I; Brautbar, C; Kwon, OJ; Brenner, T; Arnon, R; Sela, M. Direct binding of myelin basic protein and synthetic copolymer 1 to class II major histocompatibility complex molecules on living antigen-presenting cells: specificity and promiscuity. *Proc. Natl. Acad. Sci. USA*, 1994, 91, 4872-4876.

[82] Teitelbaum, D; Fridkis-Hareli, M; Arnon, R; Sela, M. Copolymer 1 inhibits chronic relapsing experimental allergic encephalomyelitis induced by proteolipid protein (PLP) peptides in mice and interferes with PLP-specific T cell responses. *J. Neuroimmunol.*, 1996, 64, 209-217.

[83] Ben-Nun, A; Mendel, I; Bakimer, R; Fridkis-Hareli, M; Teitelbaum, D; Arnon, R; Sela, M; Kerlero de Rosbo, N. The autoimmune reactivity to myelin oligodendrocyte glycoprotein (MOG) in multiple sclerosis is potentially pathogenic: effect of copolymer 1 on MOG-induced disease. *J. Neurol.*, 1996, 243 (4 Suppl 1), S14-22.

[84] Fridkis-Hareli, M; Teitelbaum, D; Arnon, R; Sela, M. Synthetic copolymer 1 and myelin basic protein do not require processing prior to binding to class II major histocompatibility complex molecules on living antigen-presenting cells. *Cell. Immunol.*, 1995, 163, 229-236.

[85] Fridkis-Hareli, M; Teitelbaum, D; Pecht, I; Arnon, R; Sela, M. Binding of copolymer 1 and myelin basic protein leads to clustering of class II MHC molecules on antigen-presenting cells. *Int. Immunol.*, 1997, 9, 925-934.

[86] Fridkis-Hareli, M; Strominger, JL. Promiscuous binding of synthetic copolymer 1 to purified HLA-DR molecules. *J. Immunol.*, 1998, 160, 4386-4397.

[87] Fridkis-Hareli, M; Neveu, JM; Robinson, RA; Lane, WS; Gauthier, L; Wucherpfennig, KW; Sela, M; Strominger, JL. Binding motifs of copolymer 1 to multiple sclerosis- and rheumatoid arthritis-associated HLA-DR molecules. *J. Immunol.*, 1999, 162, 4697-4704.

[88] Fridkis-Hareli, M; Rosloniec, EF; Fugger, L; Strominger, JL. Synthetic peptides that inhibit binding of the collagen type II 261-273 epitope to rheumatoid arthritis-associated HLA-DR1 and -DR4 molecules and collagen-specific T-cell responses. *Hum. Immunol.*, 2000, 61, 640-650.

[89] Aharoni, R; Teitelbaum, D; Arnon, R; Sela, M. Copolymer 1 acts against the immunodominant epitope 82-100 of myelin basic protein by T cell receptor antagonism in addition to major histocompatibility complex blocking. *Proc. Natl. Acad. Sci. USA*, 1999, 96, 634-639.

[90] Gran, B; Tranquill, LR; Chen, M; Bielekova, B; Zhou, W; Dhib-Jalbut, S; Martin, R. Mechanisms of immunomodulation by glatiramer acetate. *Neurology*, 2000, 55, 1704-1714.

[91] Neuhaus, O; Farina, C; Yassouridis, A; Wiendl, H; Then Bergh, F; Dose, T; Wekerle, H; Hohlfeld R. Multiple sclerosis: comparison of copolymer-1- reactive T cell lines from treated and untreated subjects reveals cytokine shift from T helper 1 to T helper 2 cells. *Proc. Natl. Acad. Sci. USA*, 2000, 97, 7452-7457.

[92] Aharoni, R; Teitelbaum, D; Arnon, R. T suppressor hybridomas and interleukin-2-dependent lines induced by copolymer 1 or by spinal cord homogenate down-regulate experimental allergic encephalomyelitis. *Eur. J. Immunol.*, 1993, 23, 17-25.

[93] Aharoni, R; Teitelbaum, D; Sela, M; Arnon, R. Copolymer 1 induces T cells of the T helper type 2 that crossreact with myelin basic protein and suppress experimental autoimmune encephalomyelitis. *Proc. Natl. Acad. Sci. USA*, 1997, 94, 10821-10826.

[94] Aharoni, R; Teitelbaum, D; Sela, M; Arnon, R. Bystander suppression of experimental autoimmune encephalomyelitis by T cell lines and clones of the Th2 type induced by copolymer 1. *J. Neuroimmunol.*, 1998, 91, 135-146.

[95] Fridkis-Hareli, M; Rosloniec, EF; Fugger, L; Strominger, JL. Synthetic amino acid copolymers that bind to HLA-DR proteins and inhibit type II collagen-reactive T cell clones. *Proc. Natl. Acad. Sci. USA*, 1998, 95, 12528-12531.

[96] Fridkis-Hareli, M; Stern, JN; Fugger, L; Strominger, JL. Synthetic peptides that inhibit binding of the myelin basic protein 85-99 epitope to multiple sclerosis-associated HLA-DR2 molecules and MBP-specific T-cell responses. *Hum. Immunol.*, 2001, 62, 753-763.

[97] Stern, JN; Illes, Z; Reddy, J; Keskin, DB;, Fridkis-Hareli, M; Kuchroo, VK; Strominger, JL. Peptide 15-mers of defined sequence that substitute for random amino acid copolymers in amelioration of experimental autoimmune encephalomyelitis. *Proc. Natl. Acad. Sci. USA*, 2005, 102, 1620-1625.

[98] Fridkis-Hareli, M; Aharoni, R; Teitelbaum, D; Arnon, R; Sela, M; Strominger, JL. Binding of random copolymers of three amino acids to class II MHC molecules. *Int. Immunol.*, 1999, 11, 635-641.

[99] Fridkis-Hareli, M; Santambrogio, L; Stern, JN; Fugger, L; Brosnan, C; Strominger, JL. Novel synthetic amino acid copolymers that inhibit autoantigen-specific T cell responses and suppress experimental autoimmune encephalomyelitis. *J. Clin. Invest.*, 2002, 109, 1635-1643.

[100] Stern, JN; Illes, Z; Reddy, J; Keskin, DB; Sheu, E; Fridkis-Hareli, M; Nishimura, H; Brosnan, CF; Santambrogio, L; Kuchroo, VK; Strominger, JL. Amelioration of proteolipid protein 139-151-induced encephalomyelitis in SJL mice by modified amino acid copolymers and their mechanisms. *Proc. Natl. Acad. Sci. USA*, 2004, 101, 11743-11748.

[101] Cocco E, Marchi P, Sardu C, Russo P, Paolillo A, Mascia MG, Solla M, Frau J, Lorefice L, Massole S, Floris G, Marrosu MG. Mitoxantrone treatment in patients with early relapsing-remitting multiple sclerosis. *Mult. Scler.*, 2007 (in press).

[102] Cartwright, MS; Jeffery, DR; Lewis, ZT; Koty, PP; Stewart, WT; Molnar, I. Mitoxantrone for multiple sclerosis causing acute lymphoblastic leukemia. *Neurology*, 2007, 68, 1630-1631.

[103] Boggild, M. Rationale and experience with combination therapies in multiple sclerosis. *J. Neurol.*, 2006, 253(Suppl 6), VI/45–VI/51.

[104] Tullman, MJ; Lublin, FD. Combination therapy in multiple sclerosis. *Curr. Neurol. Neurosci. Rep.*, 2005, 5, 245–248.

[105] Niino, M; Bodner, C; Simard, ML; *et al.* Natalizumab effects on immune cell responses in multiple sclerosis. *Ann. Neurol.*, 2006, 59, 748–754.

[106] Stuve, O; Marra, CM; Bar-Or, A; *et al.* Altered $CD4^{+}/CD8^{+}$ T-cell ratios in cerebrospinal fluid of natalizumab-treated patients with multiple sclerosis. *Arch. Neurol.*, 2006, 63, 1383–1387.

[107] Stuve, O; Marra, CM; Jerome, KR; *et al.* Immune surveillance in multiple sclerosis patients treated with natalizumab. *Ann. Neurol.*, 2006, 59, 743–747.

[108] Miller, DH; Khan, OA; Sheremata, WA; *et al.* A controlled trial of natalizumab for relapsing multiple sclerosis. *N. Engl. J. Med.*, 2003, 348, 15–23.

[109] Yousry, TA; Major, EO; Ryschkewitsch, C; *et al.* Evaluation of patients treated with natalizumab for progressive multifocal leukoencephalopathy. *N. Engl. J. Med.*, 2006, 354, 924–933.

[110] Department of Health and Human Services. Tysabri® risk minimization action plan: summary of TOUCHTM. Rockville, MD: Department of Health and Human Services; 2007.

[111] Hemmer, B; Frohman, E; Hartung, HP; Stuve, O. Central nervous system infections: a potential complication of systemic immunotherapy. *Curr. Opin. Neurol.*, 2006, 19, 271–276.

[112] Ransohoff, RM. Natalizumab and PML. *Nat. Neurosci.*, 2005, 8, 1275.

[113] Koralnik, IJ. Progressive multifocal leukoencephalopathy revisited: has the disease outgrown its name? *Ann. Neurol.*, 2006, 60, 162–173.

[114] Stuve, O; Marra, CM; Cravens, PD; *et al.* Potential risk of progressive multifocal leukoencephalopathy with natalizumab therapy: possible interventions. *Arch. Neurol.*, 2007, 64, 169–176.

[115] Reid, JL. Pharmacokinetic and pharmacodynamic aspects of the choice of components of combination therapy. *J. Hum. Hypertens.*, 1995, 9(Suppl 4), S19–S23.

[116] Toews, ML; Bylund, DB. Pharmacologic principles for combination therapy. *Proc. Am. Thorac. Soc.*, 2005, 2, 282–289.

[117] Ramtahal, J; Jacob, A; Das, K; Boggild, M. Sequential maintenance treatment with glatiramer acetate after mitoxantrone is safe and can limit exposure to immunosuppression in very active, relapsing remitting multiple sclerosis. *J. Neurol.*, 2006, 253, 1160–1164.

[118] Lublin, F; Cutter, G; Elfront, R; *et al.* A trial to assess the safety of combining interferon beta-1α and glatiramer acetate in patients with relapsing MS. *Neurology*, 2001, 56(Suppl 3), A148.

[119] Calabresi, PA; Wilterdink, JL; Rogó, JM; *et al.* An open-label trial of combination therapy with interferon beta 1α and oral methotrexate in MS. *Neurology*, 2002, 58, 314–317.

[120] Cohen, J; Antel, J; Calabresi, P; *et al.* Rational and design of the Avonex combination trial. *Mult. Scler.*, 2003, 9(Suppl 1), S139.

[121] Ubogu, EE; Cossoy, MB; Ransohoff, RM. The expression and function of chemokines involved in CNS inflammation. *Trends Pharmacol. Sci.*, 2006, 27, 48–55.

[122] Wells, TN; Power, CA; Shaw, JP; Proudfoot, AE. Chemokine blockers: therapeutics in the making? *Trends Pharmacol. Sci.*, 2006, 27, 41–47.

[123] Elices, MJ. BX-471 Berlex. *Curr. Opin. Investig. Drugs*, 2002, 3, 865–869.

[124] Zipp, F; Hartung, HP; Hillert, J; *et al.* Blockade of chemokine signaling in patients with multiple sclerosis. *Neurology*, 2006, 67, 1880–1883.

[125] Charo, IF; Ransohoff, RM. The many roles of chemokines and chemokine receptors in inflammation. *N. Engl. J. Med.*, 2006, 354, 610–621.

[126] Brinkmann, V. FTY720: mechanism of action and potential benefit in organ transplantation. *Yonsei Med. J.*, 2004, 45, 991–997.

[127] Chiba, K. FTY720, a new class of immunomodulator, inhibits lymphocyte egress from secondary lymphoid tissues and thymus by agonistic activity at sphingosine 1-phosphate receptors. *Pharmacol. Ther.*, 2005, 108, 308–319.

[128] Habicht, A; Clarkson, MR; Yang, J; *et al.* Novel insights into the mechanism of action of FTY720 in a transgenic model of allograft rejection: implications for therapy of chronic rejection. *J. Immunol.*, 2006, 176, 36–42.

[129] Matloubian, M; Lo, CG; Cinamon, G; *et al.* Lymphocyte egress from thymus and peripheral lymphoid organs is dependent on S1P receptor 1. *Nature*, 2004, 427, 355–360.

[130] Rosen, H; Goetzl, EJ. Sphingosine 1-phosphate and its receptors: an autocrine and paracrine network. *Nat. Rev. Immunol.*, 2005, 5, 560–570.

[131] Budde, K; Schmouder, RL; Brunkhorst, R; *et al.* First human trial of FTY720, a novel immunomodulator, in stable renal transplant patients. *J. Am. Soc. Nephrol.*, 2002, 13, 1073–1083.

[132] Fujino, M; Funeshima, N; Kitazawa, Y; *et al.* Amelioration of experimental autoimmune encephalomyelitis in Lewis rats by FTY720 treatment. *J. Pharmacol. Exp. Ther.*, 2003, 305, 70–77.

[133] Webb, M; Tham, CS; Lin, FF; *et al.* Sphingosine 1-phosphate receptor agonists attenuate relapsing-remitting experimental autoimmune encephalitis in SJL mice. *J. Neuroimmunol.*, 2004, 153, 108–121.

[134] Kappos, L; Antel, J; Comi, G; *et al.* Oral fingolimod (FTY720) for relapsing multiple sclerosis. *N. Engl. J. Med.*, 2006, 355, 1124–1140.

[135] Monson, NL; Cravens, PD; Frohman, EM; Hawker, K; Racke, MK. Effect of Rituximab on the Peripheral Blood and Cerebrospinal Fluid B Cells in Patients With Primary Progressive Multiple Sclerosis. *Arch. Neurol.*, 2005, 62, 258-264.

[136] Teitelbaum, D; Milo, R; Arnon, R; Sela, M. Synthetic copolymer 1 inhibits human T-cell lines specific for myelin basic protein. *Proc. Natl. Acad. Sci. USA*, 1992, 89, 137-141, 1992.

[137] Arnon, R. The development of Cop 1 (Copaxone), an innovative drug for the treatment of multiple sclerosis: personal reflections. *Immunol. Lett.*, 1996, 50, 1-15.

[138] Qin, Y; Zhang, DQ; Prat, A; Pouly, S; Antel, J. Characterization of T cell lines derived from glatiramer-acetate-treated multiple sclerosis patients. *J. Neuroimmunol.*, 2000, 108, 201-206.

[139] Duda, PW; Schmied, MC; Cook, SL; Krieger, JI; Hafler, DA. Glatiramer acetate (Copaxone) induces degenerate, Th2-polarized immune responses in patients with multiple sclerosis. *J. Clin. Invest.*, 2000, 105, 967-976.

[140] Farina, C; Then Bergh, F; Albrecht, H; Meinl, E; Yassouridis, A; Neuhaus, O; Hohlfeld, R. Treatment of multiple sclerosis with Copaxone (COP): Elispot assay

detects COP-induced interleukin-4 and interferon-gamma response in blood cells. *Brain*, 2001, 124, 705-719.

[141] Gran, B; Tranquill, LR; Chen, M; Bielekova, B; Zhou, W; Dhib-Jalbut, S; Martin, R. Mechanisms of immunomodulation by glatiramer acetate. *Neurology*, 2000, 55, 1704-1714.

[142] Kim, HJ; Ifergan, I; Antel, JP; Seguin, R; Duddy, M; Lapierre, Y; Jalili, F; Bar-Or, A. Type 2 monocyte and microglia differentiation mediated by glatiramer acetate therapy in patients with multiple sclerosis. *J. Immunol.*, 2004, 172, 7144-7153.

[143] Weber, MS; Starck, M; Wagenpfeil, S; Meinl, E; Hohlfeld, R; Farina, C. Multiple sclerosis: glatiramer acetate inhibits monocyte reactivity in vitro and in vivo. *Brain*, 2004, 127, 1370-1378.

[144] Marmont, AM. Will hematopoietic stem cell transplantation cure autoimmune diseases? *J. Autoimmun.*, 2008, 30, 145-150.

In: Stem Cell Therapy and Uses in Medical Treatment
Editor: Prasad S. Koka, pp. 65-77
ISBN: 978-1-61324-008-3

Chapter 4

Stem Cell Transplantation Modulates mRNA Gene Expression Profile in Doxorubicin-Induced Cardiomyopathy

Jens Garbade*[*1], Andreas Schubert[1#], Markus Jan Barten[1°], Heike Aupperle[2], Mani Arsalan[1], Michael A. Borger[1], Stefan Jacobs[1], Stefan Dhein[1] and Friedrich-Wilhelm Mohr[1]

[1]Dept. of Cardiac Surgery, Heart Center Leipzig, University of Leipzig, Germany,
[2]Institute of Veterinary Pathology, University of Leipzig, Faculty of Veterinary Medicine, Germany
°Moved to: Department of Cardiothoracic Surgery, Friedrich-Schiller-University, Jena, Germany

Abstract

We previously reported that epimyocardial injection of bone marrow-derived stem cells (BMCS) inhibits cardiac remodeling and prevents further functional impairment measured 28 days after cell application in doxorubicin-induced cardiomyopathic rabbit hearts. This effect could not be attributed to transdifferentiation of donor cells. We therefore speculated that paracrine actions exerted by the BMCS might play an important role in cardiac repair and functional improvement.

When transplanted locally into doxorubicin-induced cardiomyopathic rabbits, BMCS attenuate ventricular function relative to controls. The trigger of mRNA expression may be the first response to cell transplantation. However, little is known to date about the

* Corresponding author: Jens Garbade M.D. Dept. of Cardiac Surgery, Heart Center Leipzig, University of Leipzig. Struempellstr. 39. D-04289 Leipzig. Germany. Tel: +49-341-8651420. e-mail: garbade@med.uni-leipzig.de

# Who contributed equally to the study

impact of these cells on regulation of cardiomyocyte mRNA expression. In the current study we demonstrate that locally transplanted BMCS inhibit the doxorubicin-induced altered mRNA profiles and trigger reverse myocardial remodeling. Support for our hypothesis of a BMCS paracrine action is provided by globally enhanced mRNA expression of cardioprotective and pro-angiogenetic factors VEGF, bFGF and IGF.

In addition, we observed normalization of ANP mRNA levels as an indicator of improved heart function. The current study may be the first evidence that autologous BMCS may regulate gene expression profile.

Keywords: bone marrow-derived stem cell, transplantation, gene expression, myocardial regeneration, cardiomyopathy.

Introduction

Different types of adult stem cells have been proposed as a potential pool for regenerative therapy of ischemic heart disease [1-4]. Initial experimental results have displayed the same therapeutic potential in non-ischemic cardiomyopathy [5-7]. The multipotency, low immunogenicity and amenability of bone marrow-derived stem cells (BMCS) make them particularly suitable for this purpose [8]. Several groups have reported that cell transplantation in non-ischemic heart disease attenuates impaired left ventricular function [5-7]. However, the mechanisms behind this observation have not been clearly defined.

The in situ transdifferentiation of BMCS into cardiomyocytes or endothelial cells has been proposed as the mode of left ventricular functional improvement by some authors [3,4]. However, there is much debate over the probability and frequency of this phenomenon [9,10]. It has also been proposed that BMCS release angiogenic factors, regulate apoptotic cell death, induce proliferation of host cardiomyocytes, and recruit resident cardiac stem cells [11-16]. Regardless of the variety of discussed mechanisms, there appears to be agreement that stem cell application has the potential to attenuate cardiac remodeling.

We previously reported that the epimyocardial transplantation of BMCS leads to restoration of myocardial function and prevention of ventricular remodeling. Additionally, we observed an upregulation of capillary density, diminished collagen content and improved sympathoadrenal dysregulation [17,18]. However, we were unable to demonstrate the transdifferentiation of transplanted BMCS into cardiomyocytes [17,18].

In the current study, we attempted to gain insight into the potential mechanisms underlying the therapeutic properties of BMCS transplantation, with a particular focus on possible paracrine effects. We therefore investigated mRNA expression profile of various angiogenic and cardioprotective genes in remote myocardium (i.e. distant from the cell application area) in a rabbit model of doxorubicin-induced heart failure.

Materials and Methods

All experiments were conducted in accordance with guidelines published in the Guide for the Care and Use of Laboratory Animals (NIH Publication No. 85-23, revised 1996) and under protocols approved by the Institutional Animal Care and Use Committee at Leipzig University and local government authorities (Reg.-Nr.: 24-9168.11-11/03).

Animal Experiments and Study Design

Our experimental protocol has been previously published [17,18]. Briefly, heart failure was induced in three month old male White New Zealand rabbits by injection of doxorubicin (3mg/kg once a week intravenously for 6 weeks). The animals were assigned to receive either BMCS transplantation (BMCS-group, received 1.5-2.0x10^6 autologous bone marrow-derived stem cells, n=15), sham surgery (Medium-group, n=10), or no surgical therapy (Dox-group, n=6). In addition, a group of healthy rabbits without doxorubicin injections were included as controls (Control-group, n=10).

Isolation, Expansion and Labeling of Stem Cells

To avoid immune rejection, animals received autologous BMCS. Four days befor transplantation a femoral bone marrow aspirate was performed aseptically from the right hindlimb. The animals received intramuscular ketamine (50 mg/kg) and xylazine (5 mg/kg) prior to this procedure.

Bone marrow aspirate was flushed with PBS-EDTA (phosphate buffer saline, pH 7.4, EDTA 2 mM) to obtain a maximum amount of cells. The BMCS were fractionated over 1.073 g/ml Ficoll solution (Sigma, Germany) and the mononuclear cells were obtained according to the technique described by Tomita [4]. After two washing steps BMCS were resuspended in 12 ml Dulbecco`s Modified Eagel Medium (DMEM, Sigma) by adding 10% fetal bovine serum, 100 U/ml penicillin G, 100 µg/ml streptomycin (Sigma). To induce differentiation, cells were cultured with 10 µM 5-azacytidine for 24 hours (Sigma) and seeded on gelatine-coated Petri dishes and cultured at 37° C in a 5% CO2- humidified atmosphere. Cultured cells were tested to ensure freedom from Mycoplasma contamination.

The nonadherent hematopoietic cells were discarded with the medium changes, which were performed every 2 days (twice). Prior to cell transplantation, adherent cells were detached with trypsin-EDTA, passaged and labeled with 2.5µL/ml Vybrant DiI cell-labeling solution (Molecular Probes) for 30 minutes protected from light at 37°C followed by 3 washes with PBS. Cells passaged twice were harvested and used for cell transplantation. The BMCS were characterized by cell surface markers using flow cytometry (Becton Dickinson FACS Calibur System) with antibodies against CD34, CD45, CD133 (Miltenyi Biotecy, Germany) according to the manufacturer´s protocol.

Cell Transplantation

Two weeks after ending doxorubicin administration, the cardiomyopathic animals were assigned to receive either transplanted cells (BMCS-group; n = 15), transplanted medium (Medium-group; n = 10) or no surgical therapy (Dox-group; n =6). The animals were premedicated with intramuscular ketamine (50 mg/kg) and xylazine (5 mg/kg), endotracheally intubated and mechanically ventilated. Anesthesia was maintained with 2% isoflurane. A left thoracotomy through the intercostal space was performed and the left ventricle was exposed. Thereafter, the free lateral wall of the LV was identified and either 1.5-2.0*10^6 cells/mL or media (1 mL) was injected at four locations in a circular manner with a tuberculin syringe within 2 minutes. A thorax drain was inserted before the chest was closed in layers. The rabbits recovered from the surgical procedure and were treated with antibiotics and analgesics up to 72 hours postoperatively as required.

Assay of VEGF, bFGF, IGF and ANP mRNA Profile

The mRNA expression encoding for different marker genes (VEGF, bFGF, IGF and ANP) were measured 28 days postoperatively using real-time PCR. Myocardial samples (~1g) for mRNA quantification were obtained from the free wall of left ventricle (LV – outside of cell injection), the middle of interventricular septum and the free wall of right ventricle (RV). All sample sites were remote from cell transplantation application (n=6 each).

We assessed vascular endothelial growth factor (VEGF) mRNA, because of its known association with angiogenesis. Basic fibroblast growth factor (bFGF) mRNA and insulin growth factor (IGF) were quantified as a measure of angiogenesis, as well as their cardioprotective properties. In addition, we measured atrial natriuretic peptide (ANP) mRNA levels because of its association with global heart function.

The myocardial specimens were snap-frozen in liquid nitrogen immediately after final examination and stored at -80°C for mRNA analysis. Frozen tissue samples of all three compartments (LV, RV and septum, n = 6 each) were prepared with an Ultra-Turrax (IKA, Wilmington, NC) using Trizol Reagent (Invitrogen, Karlsruhe, Germany). An aliquot of total RNA (500ng) was reversely transcribed into cDNA using a Sensiscript Kit (Qiagen, Hilden, Germany) and random primers (Invitrogen) according to the instructions of manufacturers. To quantify mRNA expression levels, an aliquot of the cDNA was used in real-time PCR containing the gene-specific primers and LightCycler-FastStart DNA Master SYBR-Green I reaction mix (Roche Diagnostics, Mannheim, Germany). The specific expression levels were analyzed using LightCycler software and expressed in relation to the individual 18S rRNA intensity in relative units. Every PCR was performed 3 times, resulting in a variability of less than 10%. The used primers and PCR conditions are described in Table 1.

Statistical Anaylsis

All data are expressed as mean ± SEM throughout the manuscript. Statistical significance was analyzed by unpaired two-tailed Student′s t-test or, if appropriate, by repeated measures ANOVA followed by Bonferroni corrections for multiple comparisons. Results were considered statistically significant at a level of $p < 0.05$. All data analyses were performed using SAS software, version 6.11 (SAS Institute, Cary, NC, USA).

Results

In order to explain the potential effects of BMCS on mRNA levels we determined the regulation of various cytoprotective and angiogenic gene factors remote from epimyocardial cell transplantation.

Table 1. Characteristic and Sequences of the Used Primers

	Primersequenz	*Annealing Temperature*	*Fragment Length*	*PCR cycles*
VEGF sense	GGAGACAATAAACCCCACGA	58°C		
VEGF antisense	CACACTCCAGGCTTTCATCA	58°C	188 bp	40
b-FGF sense	GGTTTCTTCCTGCGTATCCA	58°C		
b-FGF antisense	ACTGCCCAGTTCGTTTCAGT	58°C	286 bp	40
IGF sense	TGGATGCTCTTCAGTTCGTG	58°C		
IGF antisense	TTGTTTCCTGCACTCCCTCT	58°C	271 bp	40
ANP sense	AAGAAGCAGCTAACGGCACA	58°C		
ANP antisense	CATCAGATCTGCGTTGGACA	58°C	155 bp	40
18SrRNA sense	AAACGGCTACCACATCCAAG	58°C		
18SrRNA antisense	CTACGCACCCTCCACAAGAT	60°C	259 bp	21

Therefore we measured VEGF, bFGF, IGF and ANP mRNA values in myocardial samples (n=6, each group) from the LV (outside of cell injection area), the septum and the RV.

In general, chronic doxorubicin administration resulted in a significant upregulation of VEGF, bFGF and IGF mRNA in the LV and the RV compared to the healthy Control-group (Figure 1-3). In the interventricular septum (Dox-group vs. Control-group), the differences for bFGF and IGF mRNA levels failed to reach statistical significance (Figure 2 and 3).

Interestingly, the mRNA of ANP was also increased in the Dox-group vs. Control-group (Figure 4). The increase in ANP mRNA is presumably secondary to the observed impaired heart function, as previously described [17,18].

The mRNA expression profile of VEGF, bFGF and IGF in all three myocardial regions in the BMCS-group vs. Medium-group are illustrated in Figures 1-3. The mRNA levels of VEGF, bFGF and IGF were significantly increased in the BMCS-treated group in the RV and septum, but failed to reach statistical significance in the LV.

The mRNA levels of ANP revealed a significant downregulation in the BMCS-group when compared to Medium-treated rabbits (Figure 4). BMCS transplantation resulted in an ANP mRNA level that was not significantly different from the healthy control animals (Figure 4).

Additionally, the mRNA levels for all analyzed genes were slightly higher in the Dox-group vs. Medium-group, except for ANP.

By histological investigation, we found vastly areas of replacement fibrosis or foci of degenerative myocardium made of vacuolated degenerative myocytes were also presented. These morphological alterations are characteristics of this non-ischemic heart failure rabbit model. The observed histology was not attributed to the locally injections or the presence or absence of BMCS (Figure 5B and C).

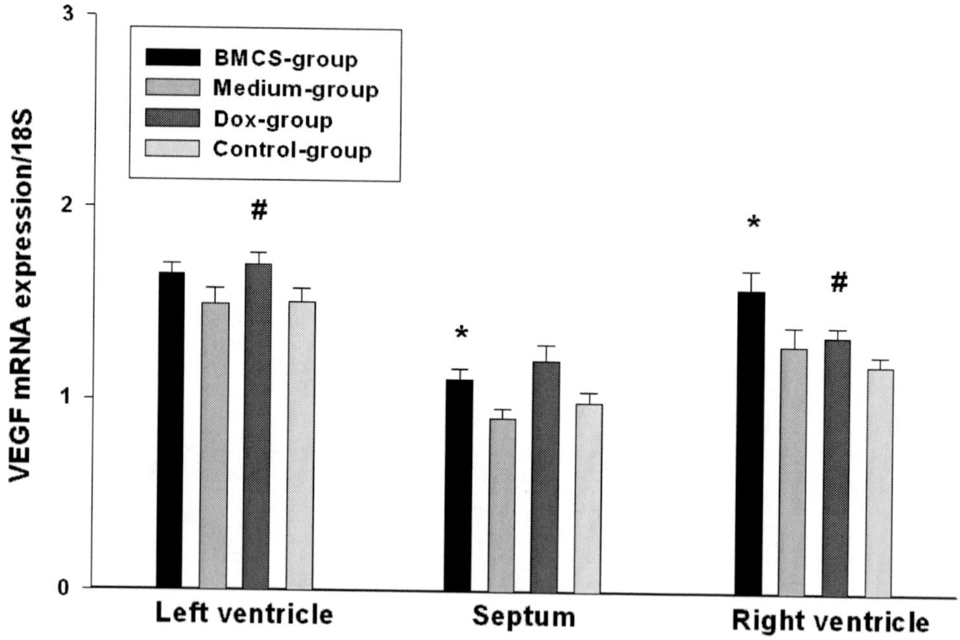

Figure 1. VEGF mRNA expression from LV, septum and RV myocardial samples (n=6, each group). The mRNA´s in the BMCS-treated group were upregulated when compared to the Medium-group ($^{*}p<0.05$ vs. Medium-group). There was higher VEGF mRNA expression in the Dox-group vs. Control-group ($^{\#}p<0.05$). Data are shown as mean±SEM.

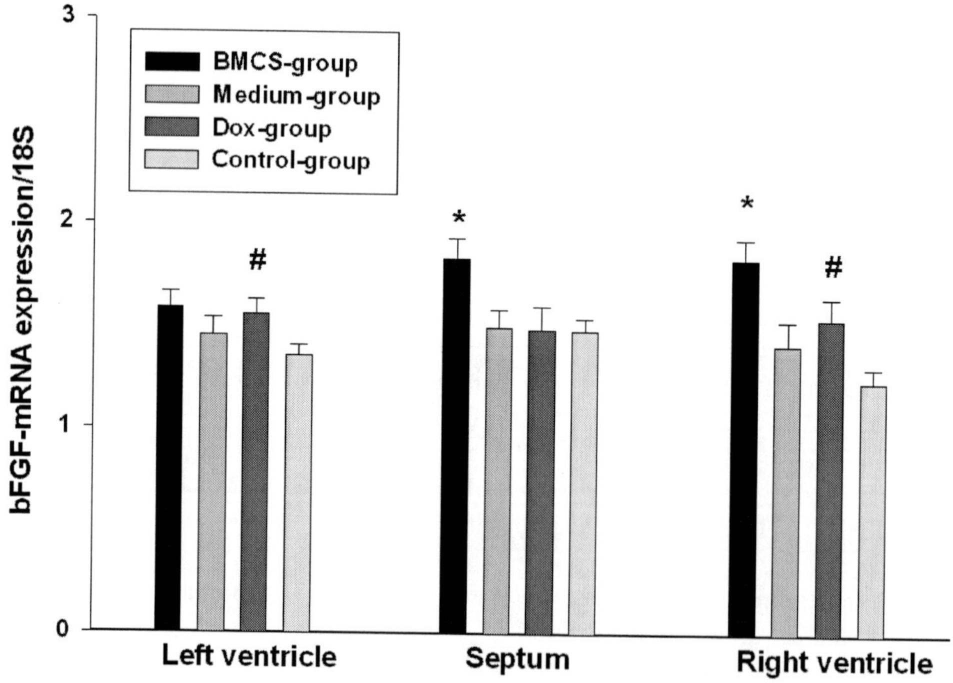

Figure 2. bFGF mRNA expression from LV, septum and RV myocardial samples (n=6, each group). The bFGF mRNA´s in the BMCS-treated group were upregulated when compared to the Medium-group ($^{*}p<0.05$ vs. Medium-group). There was higher bFGF mRNA expression in the Dox-group vs. Control-group ($^{\#}p<0.05$). Data are shown as mean±SEM.

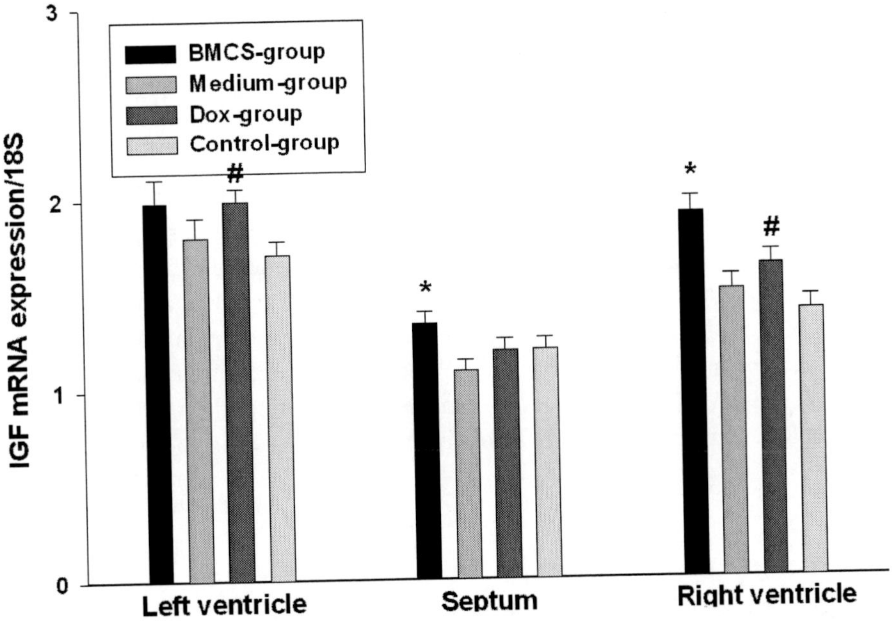

Figure 3. IGF mRNA expression from LV, septum and RV myocardial samples (n=6, each group). There was a higher expression profile of IGF mRNA's in the BMCS–group compared to Medium-group and Dox-group vs. Control-group ($^{*}p<0.05$ vs. Medium-group and $^{\#}p<0.05$ Dox- vs. Control-group). Data are shown as mean±SEM.

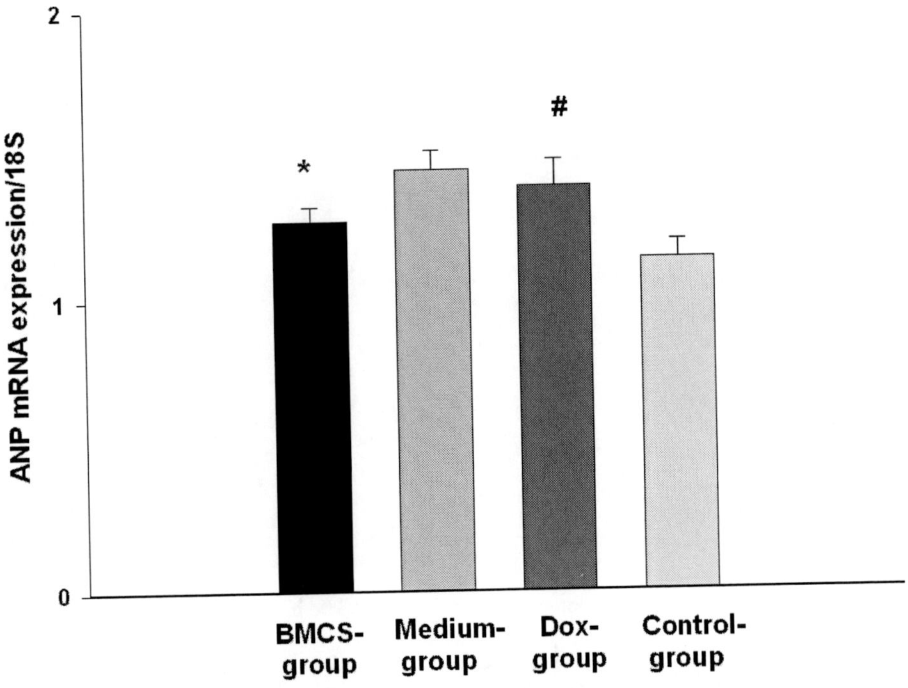

Figure 4. ANP mRNA expression (n=6, each group). The mRNA ANP level of the BMCS-group nearly reached the level of healthy controls and was significantly different from the Medium-group ($^{*}p<0.05$). The ANP mRNA was significantly higher in the Dox-group compared to Control-group ($^{\#}p<0.05$). Data are shown as mean±SEM.

Under fluorescence microscopy, we observed only a few transplanted cells/visual field and mostly remnants showing Vybrand DiI red fluorescence, in BMCS treated hearts in the vicinity of the injection sites, but not in the sham-operated hearts (Figure 5D). We did not observe transplanted cells remote from cell application in the LV, but only in the area of cell injection. We also observed red fluorescent detritus in these areas. At the cell injection site, we found a fibrotic scar in both the BMCS- and Medium-group (Fig. 5B and C). Stem cells could not be identified in HE stained slides. Using fluorescence microscopy, single large cells with oval nuclei showing a specific intracytoplasmic signal derived from DiI loading in the sites of stem cell injection were observed. From the morphology, it was unclear whether these cells were original BMCS or macrophages with phagocytosed remnants of BMCS (Figure 5D). In the sites of medium injection, no cells with a specific intracytoplasmic signal were identified. We observed no evidence of transplanted cell migration to the interventricular septum or theRV. Furthermore, no DiI positive cells were seen in the liver, spleen or other organs.

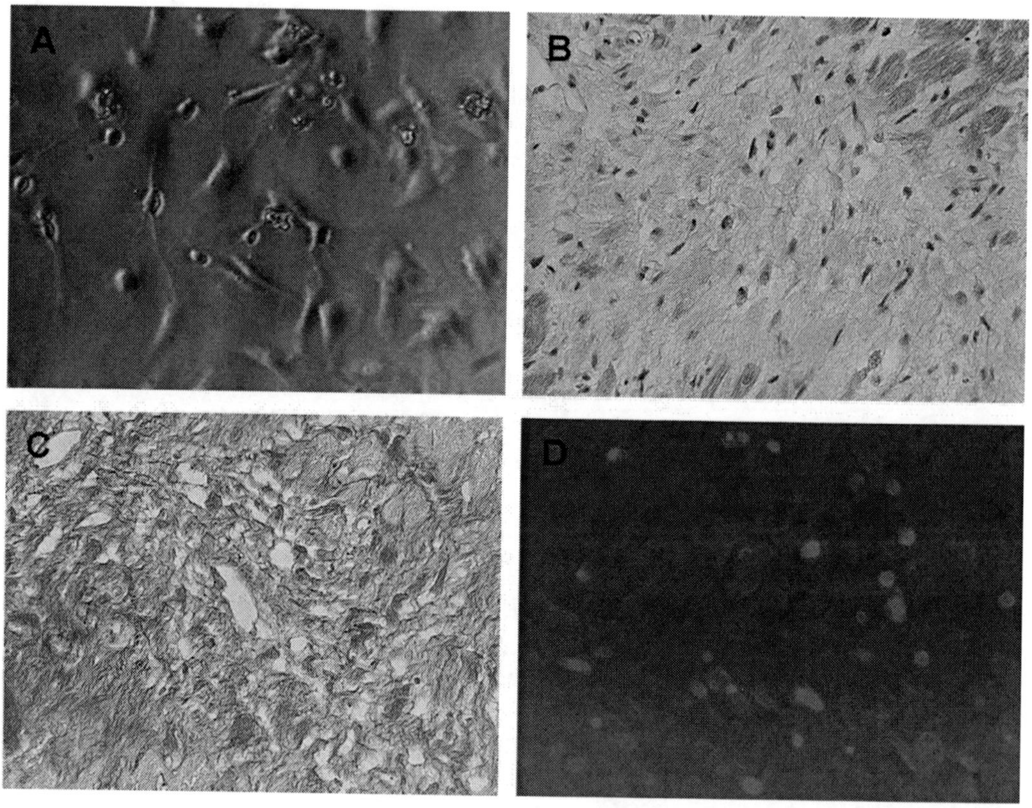

Figure 5. (A): Bone marrow-derived stem cells in-vitro culture. The majority of cultured cells were spindle-like cells after 4 days of culture and purification (magnification: x400). (B and C): The injection site (BMCS-group) is characterized by focal fibroblastic epicarditis spreading into the surrounding myocardium (B: H&E and C: Picrosirius red stain, magnification: x200). (D): Transplanted red fluorescent cells and red fluorescing detritius are shown (DiI-staining), which were found only in the injection site (magnification: x200).

Additionally, the FACS-analysis for clearly characterisation of transplanted cells failed due to incompetent antibodies in our rabbit-model.

Discussion

We previously demonstrated that epimyocardial transplantation of BMCS results in improved left ventricular function in doxorubicin-induced cardiomyopathy [17,18]. In the current study, we provided some mechanistic insights into the action of BMCS transplantation. We demonstrated that BMCS regulate the mRNA gene expression of cardiac tissue cytokines. We also showed that local epimyocardial cell application significantly regulates the mRNA profiles in remote tissue, i.e. away from the cell injection site. These new data reinforce the recent observations of cardioprotective and pro-angiogenic properties of BMCS transplantation and may support the hypothesis that such effects are the result of paracrine mechanisms.

The paracrine hypothesis is further supported by the fact that we found no evidence for BMCS transdifferentiation into cardiomyocytes and no migration of the locally injected cells [17,18].

We used the pretreatment of BMCS with 5-azacytidine (10 μM) for 24 hours in-vitro to push the transdifferantiation into cardiac lineage. Previously, we observed that the environment (co-culture with spontaneous beating cells, the supernatant of beating heart cells) and the incubation with 5-azacytidine supports the development into cardiac lineage of BMCS. The expression of β-MHC and β1-adrenoceptor mRNA was higher in co-culture with beating heart cells or 5-azacytidine compared to mono-culture of BMCS [24].

Our method of incubation with 5-azacytidine is based on the findings by different groups. Makino et al. described for the first time that murine BMCS transdifferenіated into beating heart cells expressing cardiac phenotype when treated with 5-azacytidine [23]. Additionally, Tomita reported that the optimal concentration for cardiomyogenic differentiation is 10μM for 24 hours [4]. The mechanism by which 5-azacytidine promotes cardiomyogenic phenotype remains unclear.

In the current study, however, we could not show any evidence for transdifferentiation of transplanted cells.

We have also previously reported that BMCS transplantation leads to significantly less β-adrenoceptor down-regulation in the septum and LV of doxorubicin-treated rabbits. We therefore concluded that BMCS improve sympathoadrenal dysregulation [18]. Such regulation might be very important in the long-term remodeling process.

We have also previously reported that BMCS transplantation resulted in significantly improved contractility, as measured by invasive testing [17,18]. The downregulation and normalization of ANP mRNA following BMCS transplantation supports our previous observation.

Another point of interest is the mechanical stabilization property of stem cells and subsequent attenuation of cardiac remodelling [11]. In this regard, we observed that bone marrow cell injection into the LV resulted in marked differences of collagen content and MMP/TIMP expression in the whole heart [18].

Interestingly, the data published by Lu and colleagues focusing on the regulation of extracellular matrix in doxorubicin-treated hearts showed that bone marrow cells downregulate MMP-1 expression. The definitive underlying mechanisms, however, could be not determined [12]. It is known that the MMP-family plays a pivotal role in the regulation of extracellular matrix and cardiac remodeling.

Gnecchi et al. reported that several genes released by mesenchymal stem cells, coding for factors VEGF, FGF-2, HGF and IGF-1, are upregulated and are potential mediators of cardiac regeneration exerted by these cells [15]. A recent study by Fazel et al. utilizing chimeric mice with a background mutation in the c-kit receptor shows that cells expressing c-kit are recruited from bone marrow and benefit the heart by the release of angiogenic substances [16]. Similarly, paracrine secretion from BMCS has been shown to enhance proliferation of endothelial and smooth muscle cells resulting in attenuated muscle atrophy and fibrosis in a murine hindlimb ischemia model [19].

In addition to its growth-promoting and antiapoptotic action, IGF-1 has been reported to increase cardiomyocyte contractility in vitro and to improve myocardial function [20,21].

We believe that our data emphasize the hypothesis of paracrine actions mediated by locally transplanted BMCS. We found BMCS are capable of regulating the mRNA expression profile coding for cardioprotective, pro-angiogenic and anti-apoptotic genes.

It is important to keep in mind, however, that our findings on mRNA levels are not necessarily transferable to downstream protein expression.

It is currently thought that paracrine mediators (VEGF, bFGF, IGF-1, SDF-1) secreted by BMCS might be involved in early repair of ischemic heart by preventing cardiomyocyte apoptosis and improving cardiac function [22]. However, myocardial regeneration derived from resident or circulating cardiac precursor cells attracted by factors from BMCS is another possible explanation.

We can only speculate that this might be one reason for our observed modified regulation of cardiac tissue mRNA.

Although our experiment does not provide definitive mechanistic evidence for the observed beneficial effects of BMCS transplantation, our findings on mRNA expression profile support a paracrine mechanism. We believe paracrine effects of transplanted cells on recipient cell compartments may lead to the promotion of angiogenesis, the preservation of collagen homeostasis and the modification of mRNA profiles locally and remotely. However, further studies are required.

Principle Limitations of Our Study

We did not provide a definitely characterisation of cells due to problems with the antibodies (species rabbit) and grading of engraftment. Also, we did not provide a comparison between different sources of stem cells and routes of application. Nevertheless, we mostly wanted to establish a proof of concept that locally transplanted BMCS have an effect on regulation of mRNA levels in the donor organ.

The results of the current study are in agreement with previously published papers as regards the potential improvement of function on a global non-ischemic form of heart failure. Our data indicate that the transplantation of BMCS influence the globally mRNA expression and may translate into a functional benefit in a rabbit model of dilated heart failure.

Conclusion

To the best of our knowledge, this is the first study to demonstrate modifications of global mRNA expression profiles after local transplantation of autologous BMCS in a rabbit model of doxorubicin-induced cardiomyopathy. The therapeutic benefits of these cells appear to be attributable primarily to diffusible factors released by the BMCS, acting in a paracrine regulatory loop on mRNA expression in all cardiac chambers.

Acknowledgments

This work was supported by grant of the German Heart Foundation "Deutsche Stiftung für Herzforschung" by grant F/08/03. This study could not have been performed without the dedicated support of A. Schubert for performing the mRNA analysis, K. Schneider and C. Ullmann (Experimental Laboratory Dept. Cardiac Surgery, Heart Center Leipzig, Germany), and Dr. P Madaj and P. Windgassen (Department for Experimental Animal Research, University of Leipzig, Geramany) for caring of animals and technical support.

References

[1] Dimmeler S, Zeiher AM, Schneider MD. Unchain my heart: the scientific foundations of cardiac repair. *J. Clin. Invest.* 115, 572, 2005.

[2] Bartunek J, Dimmeler S, Drexler H, Fernandez-Aviles F, Galinanes M, Janssens S, Martin J, Mathur A, Menasche P, Priori S, Strauer B, Tendera M, Wijns W, Zeiher A; task force of the European Society of Cardiology.The consensus of the task force of the European Society of Cardiology concerning the clinical investigation of the use of autologous adult stem cells for repair of the heart. *Eur. Heart J.* 27, 1338, 2006.

[3] Orlic D, Kajstura J, Chimenti S, Jakoniuk I, Anderson SM, Li B, Pickel J, McKay R, Nadal-Ginard B, Bodine DM, Leri A, Anversa P. Bone marrow cells regenerate infarcted myocardium. *Nature* 410, 702, 2001.

[4] Tomita S, Li RK, Weisel RD, Mickle DA, Kim EF, Sakai T, Jia FQ. Autologous transplantation of bone marrow cells improves damaged heart function. *Circulation* 100, 247, 1999.

[5] Nagaya N, Kangawa K, Itoh T, Iwase T, Murakami S, Miyahara Y, Fujii T, Uematsu M, Ohgushi H, Yamagishi M, Tokudome T, Mori H, Miyatake K, Kitamura S. Transplantation of mesenchymal stem cells improves cardiac function in a rat model of dilated cardiomyopathy. *Circulation* 112, 1128, 2005.

[6] Agbulut O, Menot ML, Li Z, Marotte F, Paulin D, Hagege AA, Chomienne C, Samuel JL, Menasche P. Temporal patterns of bone marrow cell differentiation following transplantation in doxorubicin-induced cardiomyopathy. *Cardiovasc Res.*58, 451, 2003.

[7] Suzuki K, Murtuza B, Suzuki N, Smolenski RT, Yacoub MH. Intracoronary infusion of skeletal myoblasts improves cardiac function in doxorubicin-induced heart failure. *Circulation* 104, I213, 2001.

[8] Pelacho B, Aranguren XL, Mazo M, Abizanda G, Gavira JJ, Clavel C, Gutierrez-Perez M, Luttun A, Verfaillie CM, Prosper F. Plasticity and cardiovascular applications of multipotent adult progenitor cells.Nat Clin Pract *Cardiovasc. Med.* 4, S15, 2007.

[9] Murry CE, Soonpaa MH, Reinecke H, Nakajima H, Nakajima HO, Rubart M, Pasumarthi KB, Virag JI, Bartelmez SH, Poppa V, Bradford G, Dowell JD, Williams DA, Field LJ. Haematopoietic stem cells do not transdifferentiate into cardiac myocytes in myocardial infarcts. *Nature* 428, 668, 2004.

[10] Balsam LB, Wagers AJ, Christensen JL, Kofidis T, Weissman IL, Robbins RC. Haematopoietic stem cells adopt mature haematopoietic fates in ischaemic myocardium. *Nature* 428, 664, 2004.

[11] Lyngbaek S, Schneider M, Hansen JL, Sheikh SP. Cardiac regeneration by resident stem and progenitor cells in the adult heart. *Basic Res. Cardiol.* 102, 101, 2007.

[12] Lu C, Arai M, Misao Y, Chen X, Wang N, Onogi H, Kobayashi H, Uno Y, Takemura G, Minatoguchi S, Fujiwara T, Fujiwara H. Autologous bone marrow cell transplantation improves left ventricular function in rabbit hearts with cardiomyopathy via myocardial regeneration-unrelated mechanisms. *Heart Vessels* 21, 180, 2006.

[13] Spinale FG, Coker ML, Heung LJ, Bond BR, Gunasinghe HR, Etoh T, Goldberg AT, Zellner JL, Crumbley AJ. A matrix metalloproteinase induction/activation system exists in the human left ventricular myocardium and is upregulated in heart failure. *Circulation* 102, 1944, 2000.

[14] Tyagi SC, Kumar S, Voelker DJ, Reddy HK, Janicki JS, Curtis JJ. Differential gene expression of extracellular matrix components in dilated cardiomyopathy. *J. Cell Biochem.* 63, 185, 1996.

[15] Gnecchi M, He H, Noiseux N, Liang OD, Zhang L, Morello F, Mu H, Melo LG, Pratt RE, Ingwall JS, Dzau VJ. Evidence supporting paracrine hypothesis for Akt-modified mesenchymal stem cell-mediated cardiac protection and functional improvement. *FASEB J.* 20, 661, 2006.

[16] Fazel S, Cimini M, Chen L, Li S, Angoulvant D, Fedak P, Verma S, Weisel RD, Keating A, Li RK. Cardioprotective c-kit+ cells are from the bone marrow and regulate the myocardial balance of angiogenic cytokines. *J. Clin. Invest* 116, 1865, 2006.

[17] Dhein S, Garbade J, Rouabah D, Abraham G, Ungemach FR, Schneider K, Ullmann C, Aupperle H, Gummert JF, Mohr FW. Effects of autologous bone marrow stem cell transplantation on beta-adrenoceptor density and electrical activation pattern in a rabbit model of non-ischemic heart failure. *J. Cardiothorac. Surg.* 26, 17, 2006.

[18] Aupperle H, Garbade J, Schubert A, Barten M, Dhein S, Schoon HA, Mohr FW. Effects of autologous stem cells on immunohistochemical patterns and gene expression of metalloproteinases and their tissue inhibitors in Doxorubicin cardiomyopathy in a rabbit model. *Vet. Pathol.* 44, 494, 2007.

[19] Kinnaird T, Stabile E, Burnett MS, Shou M, Lee CW, Barr S, Fuchs S, Epstein SE. Local delivery of marrow-derived stromal cells augments collateral perfusion through paracrine mechanisms. Circulation. 2004 Mar 30;109(12):1543-9. Epub 2004 Mar 15. Erratum in: *Circulation* 112, 73, 2005.

[20] Cittadini A, Stromer H, Katz SE, Clark R, Moses AC, Morgan JP, Douglas PS. Differential cardiac effects of growth hormone and insulin-like growth factor-1 in the rat. A combined in vivo and in vitro evaluation. *Circulation* 93, 800, 1996.

[21] Duerr RL, McKirnan MD, Gim RD, Clark RG, Chien KR, Ross J Jr. Cardiovascular effects of insulin-like growth factor-1 and growth hormone in chronic left ventricular failure in the rat. *Circulation* 93, 2188, 1996.

[22] Xu M, Uemura R, Dai Y, Wang Y, Pasha Z, Ashraf M. In vitro and in vivo effects of bone marrow stem cells on cardiac structure and function. *J. Mol. Cell Cardiol.* 42, 441, 2007.

[23] Makino S, Fukuda K, Miyoshi S, Konishi F, Kodama H, Pan J, Sano M, Takahashi T, Hori S, Abe H, Hata J, Umezawa A, Ogawa S, Cardiomyocytes can be generated from marrow stromal cells in vitro. *J. Clin. Invest.* 103:697-705, 1999.

[24] Garbade J, Schubert A, Scheffler A, Walther T, Gummert J, Dhein S, Mohr WF. Transdifferentiation and cell-fusion are two different ways of bone marrow stromal cells to develop into cardiac lineage. *Thorac. Cardiovasc. Surg.* 53, 2005.

In: Stem Cell Therapy and Uses in Medical Treatment
Editor: Prasad S. Koka, pp. 79-91
ISBN: 978-1-61324-008-3

Chapter 5

Human Somatic Cell Nuclear Transfer and Parthenogenesis: Preliminary Indian Experience

Deepa Bhartiya*[*1,2], William Ritchie[1,3], Indira Hinduja[4], Pandit Nandedkar[2], Kusum Zaveri[4], Leena Mukadam[4], Parul Chohan[2], Archana Patwardhan[2], Punam Nagvenkar[2], Neeraj Kumar[2], Pollyanna Tat[5], Nadine M Richings[5] and Paul J. Verma[5]

[1]These authors contributed equally
[2]Stem Cell Biology Department, National Institute for Research In Reproductive Health, JM Street, Mumbai, India
[3]Roslin Embryology Ltd, SC317801, Edinburgh, UK
[4]INKUS IVF Clinic, Charni Road, Mumbai, India; [5]Monash Institute of Medical Research, 27-31 Wright Street, Clayton, VIC 3168, Australia

Abstract

The aim of the present study was to conduct preliminary experiments towards generation of autologous human embryonic stem cell lines by somatic cell nuclear transfer (SCNT) and parthenogenesis. A total of fifteen MII human oocytes were obtained from six female donors from a collaborating IVF clinic. Each woman having produced more than 20 eggs, donated 2- 3 eggs for research with written informed consent. Nine oocytes were used for SCNT and six for parthenogenesis.

* Address all correspondence to: Dr Deepa Bhartiya, Assistant Director and Head, Stem Cell Biology Department, National Institute for Research In Reproductive Health, Jehangir Merwanji Street, Mumbai 400 012. India. E- mail: deepa_bhartiya@yahoo.com

For SCNT, the meiotic spindle of MII human oocytes was removed after visualization using a POLSCOPE, and the somatic cell was injected into the enucleated cytoplast, circumventing the need for electrofusion of the somatic cell and cytoplast. Six out of nine oocytes survived reconstruction during SCNT and four divided. Nuclear assessment of SCNT embryos by Hoechst 33342 staining confirmed nuclear division in some embryos post SCNT.

Parthenogenetic activation was carried out by calcium ionomycin followed by 6-DMAP treatment. All the activated eggs showed presence of pronuclei after 16 hours, four out of six oocytes showed cleavage and one embryo developed into a compacted morula. It was placed on a feeder layer but neither attached nor showed any further growth.

We believe the generation of autologous ES cell lines is essential to circumvent immune rejection if embryonic stem cells are to be used widely for therapy, however extensive standardization and optimization of technology is warranted.

Keywords: Embryonic stem cells, SCNT, parthenogenesis, POLSCOPE.

Introduction

Stem cell biology is an exciting area of science and therapeutic applications of stem cells hold great promise for medical and veterinary treatment. However, much research and discovery is required to realize this potential. Currently, India has four human embryonic stem cell (ESC) lines derived on mouse feeders [1,2] and two maintained on human feeders [3]. Research to differentiate these ESC lines to specific lineages is underway. The Government of India is committed to funding stem cell research and supporting international collaborations. To this end, a training course supported by Department of Biotechnology, Government of India was held at that National Institute for Research in Reproductive Health (NIRRH), Mumbai in December 2007. The aim of the course was to develop expertise in micro-manipulation techniques associated with somatic cell nuclear transfer (SCNT) and to create autologous embryonic stem cell lines. Further, the use of fifteen human oocytes to generate preliminary data on SCNT and parthenogenesis was approved by the NIRRH Human Ethics Committee. Nine oocytes were used for preliminary investigation of SCNT and six oocytes were chemically activated to trigger parthenogenetic development. Results of this preliminary study are documented and discussed in the light of existing status of human SCNT and parthenogenesis aimed at derivation of patient -specific ES cell lines.

Study Subjects and Methods

Human Ethics and Oocyte Donation

The NIRRH Ethics Committee approved use of fifteen human eggs for the preliminary study. The Monash University Standing Committee on Ethics in Research involving Humans (SCERH) also approved the project. All donated oocytes were obtained from donors who were enrolled for egg donation program, after granting written informed consent, from INKUS IVF Centre, a fertility center located in Mumbai that is fully compliant with Indian

ART guidelines. Oocyte donors, with at least one previous successful delivery were selected for egg donation program for reproductive purposes. The women underwent controlled ovarian hyper-stimulation. Briefly the women were superovulated by the long protocol, which included GnRH agonist (500μg subcutaneously from Day 21 of the menstrual cycle, reduced to 250 μg along with HMG) and HMG injections (225 IU intramuscular daily from Day 2 till optimal response was achieved) to induce follicular recruitment and growth. Treatment was continued until an optimal response was obtained i.e. at least 3 follicles measuring 18 mm and estradiol levels 250 pgm per developed follicle. Ovum pickup was performed 36 hours after administration of 10,000 IU of hCG, and oocyte donors producing more than 20 oocytes consensually and altruistically donated 2-3 oocytes for research.

Materials

All chemicals were purchased from Sigma-Aldrich (USA, http://www.sigmaaldrich.com) unless otherwise stated. All embryo manipulations were performed at 37°C. Culture medium was pre-incubated to 37°C and, when necessary, pre-equilibrated in a humidified atmosphere of 6% CO_2, 5% O_2, 89% N_2 in a triple-gas incubator (RS Biotech, UK).

Preparation of Karyoplast

Serum starved human male fetal fibroblasts were used for preparing the karyoplast (Fig 1c). Briefly, the fetal fibroblast cells were isolated from fetal limb muscle tissue collected after medical termination of pregnancy. The fetal fibroblast cell line was established and maintained in animal derived component free (ADCF) DME / high modified medium (Hyclone, USA) supplemented with 10% ES- certified FBS (Hyclone, USA), 1% v/v non-essential amino acids, 1% v/v 200mM glutamine (Invitrogen, USA) and 1% v/v Penicillin-Streptomycin at 37^0C and 5% CO_2. The cell lines were screened for the presence of HIV I and II, HbsAg, HCV and mycoplasma prior to their use. For preparing karyoplasts, the fetal fibroblast cell culture was maintained in 0.5% FBS (Hyclone, USA) for 5 days at 37^0C and 5% CO_2 environment. These somatic cells were harvested (0.05% Trypsin-EDTA) to a single cell suspension, washed, placed in oocyte wash buffer (Cook IVF, Australia) and kept on ice until use.

Preparation of Cytoplast and Viewing of Spindle

The cumulus cells surrounding the eggs were removed by repeated gentle pipetting in 40IU/ml hyaluronidase enzyme in IVF medium (COOK IVF, Australia) under oil. Cumulus free MII oocytes were transported to the research lab in a portable CO_2 incubator (K Systems, Denmark) within 30 minutes of collection. After equilibration for 30 minutes, they were examined for the presence of the spindle using a POLSCOPE (CRI, USA). Briefly, the oocytes were placed in the oocyte wash buffer (COOK IVF, Australia) in a glass bottom dish (WillCo Wells BV WG PLEIN 287, Netherlands), the spindle was viewed and images were captured using Oosight Ultra software. Later the oocytes were placed in cytochalasin B (5μg/ml) drops in oocyte wash buffer medium for at least 15 minutes at 37°C, prior to further processing.

Somatic Cell Nuclear Transfer

A hole was made in the zona pellucida of MII oocyte with spindle, using a laser (500 microseconds, SATURN laser with Cronus Embryo Analysis Software, Research Instruments, UK). An 18μm enucleation pipette was used to extract the spindle along with a minimal amount of cytoplasm. The extraction procedure was performed live under the POLSCOPE in most instances and completed within fraction of a minute per egg. After enucleation the cytoplasts were washed 3- 4 times in oocyte wash buffer (COOK IVF, Australia) and placed in a fresh drop of IVF culture medium (COOK IVF, Australia). The somatic cells (see above) were resuspended in a 10% PVP drop. Individual somatic cell was picked up with a 9μm ICSI needle (Humagen, USA) and injected into the cytoplast. The SCNT reconstructed oocytes were allowed sufficient time to heal at the injection site before removal from the manipulation chamber. They were later activated by treatment with 5μM calcium ionomycin in IVF medium (COOK IVF, Australia) for 5 minutes. After three washes in IVF medium, they were transferred to a fresh drop of IVF medium containing 2 mM 6-DMAP for 3-4 hour incubation under paraffin oil in an atmosphere of 6% CO_2, 5% O_2, 89% N_2. After 2-3 washes in IVF medium, they were incubated in fresh drops of IVF medium. Next day, they were checked for pronuclei and then transferred to cleavage medium. Medium was changed daily and at 6 to 8- cell stage embryos were transferred to blastocyst medium. Growth arrested embryos were stained with 5 μg/ml of Hoechst 33342 for 15 minutes at 37°C and viewed by UV2A epifluorescence microscopy.

Parthenogenesis

Six metaphase II oocytes were activated with 5μm calcium ionomycin for 5 minutes followed by 2 mM 6-DMAP for 3- 4 hours in IVF medium and cultured similar to SCNT embryos.

Embryo development and cleavage after SCNT and parthenogenesis was evaluated under an inverted microscope (NIKON TE 2000-S) with warm stage and photographed.

The morula developed following parthenogenesis was subjected to treatment with pronase to lyse the zona pellucida, washed thrice in hES cell medium and placed on mitotically inactivated human fetal fibroblast feeder as described elsewhere [3].

Results

Viewing of Eggs under POLSCOPE

The spindle of all the oocytes was easily visualized (Figure 1 A, B) using the POLSCOPE, an apparatus that measures birefringence ("Oosight", CRI, USA).

Somatic Cell Nuclear Transfer

We observed that the spindle could be removed while viewing under POLSCOPE in real time (Figure 1 D, E). A serum starved somatic cell (Figure 1 C) was inserted into the centre of the enucleated cytoplast. 6/9 eggs survived reconstruction and four of them divided (Figure 2) associated with varying degree of fragmentation.

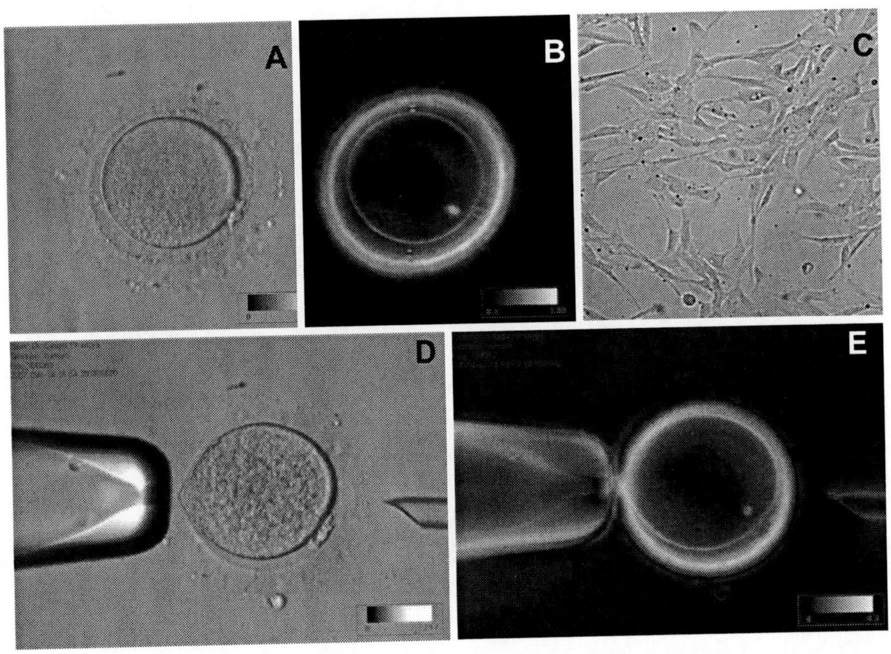

Figure 1. Human MII egg observed under inverted microscope (A) and under POLSCOPE (B). Note the presence of spindle under POLSCOE. Human fetal fibroblast used for transfer into enucleated egg (C). Procedure of spindle extraction under inverted microscope (D) and POLSCOPE (E). The meiotic spindle is extracted live while being viewed under POLSCOPE.

None of the embryos divided beyond 8 to 10 -cell stage and Hoechst 33342 staining of some of the arrested SCNT embryos confirmed nuclear division.

Parthenogenesis

Well-defined pronuclei were detected in all the eggs activated parthenogenetically. However, only 4/6 oocytes cleaved (Figure 3). Varying degrees of fragmentation was observed in the cultured embryos, which ultimately arrested in development. One of the embryos developed up to compaction (Figure 3) but did not develop further to form a blastocyst. It was placed on a feeder layer, after zona removal, to permit attachment and further proliferation, but no further growth was observed.

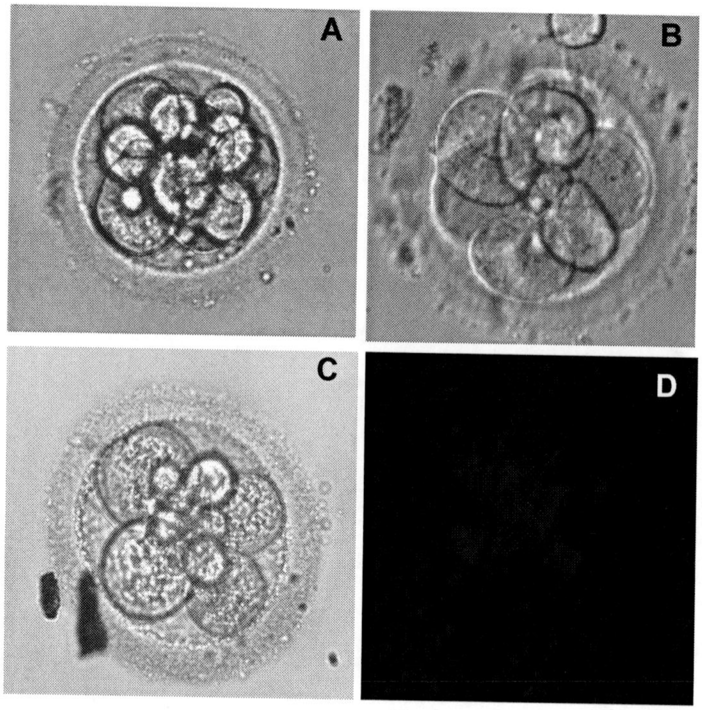

Figure 2. Embryos obtained 4- 5 days post somatic cell nuclear transfer (A- C). Hoechst staining of embryo (C) indicates nuclear division (D).

Discussion

Egg cytoplasm possesses unique capacity to reprogram adult somatic cells and revert them back to the embryonic state. These factors present in the egg, yet unidentified, bring about global epigenetic changes in the adult cell DNA whereby the genes responsible for the differentiated state are 'switched off' and embryonic genes are 'turned on'. These differential epigenetic changes of genomic DNA including methylation and histone modifications occur within 2- 3 hours post reconstruction of the eggs during the process of SCNT.

The phenomenon of induced pluripotency which involves *de novo* reprogramming of adult somatic cells to an embryonic state [4] has been hailed as potentially an ethically and technically superior alternative to SCNT for the generation of autologous embryonic stem cells. As this is a new technology, the mechanisms that result in this form of reprogramming as yet not understood, it is difficult at this stage to decide which will emerge as a better option and has been adequately reviewed elsewhere [5,6]. Regardless, there is a need for nuclear transfer embryonic stem cells to be used as a "Gold Standard' to compare reprogrammed cells against.

Successful and efficient generation of autologous human embryonic stem cell lines will revolutionize clinical management of various degenerative diseases, since it would enable embryonic stem cell therapy without the risk of immune rejection [6,7]. Although the efficiency of deriving nuclear transfer embryonic stem cell lines (20%) is significantly higher than producing a viable offspring by reproductive cloning (0.2%) in mice, the success achieved in human is minimal at present [8-13]. In addition to SCNT, autologous ES cell lines can also be derived by parthenogenetic activation of eggs and this approach has successfully resulted in the generation of pluripotent human embryonic stem cell lines [14].

Hurdles, which exist for the derivation of autologous embryonic stem cell lines are both ethical and technical. The ethical hurdle impacts on the availability of good quality M II human oocytes. It has been reported that the use of high quality oocytes (fresh M II from young donors) is necessary for successful SCNT [13]. In India, SCNT is a restricted area of research and ethical clearance from Institute Ethics Committee and then National Apex Committee will be essential to carry out SCNT. Reproductive cloning is not permitted as per ICMR-DBT guidelines for stem cell research (www.icmr.nic.in). It is generally accepted that successful derivation of autologous SCNT embryonic stem cell lines is technology based and not a biological problem *per se*. One technical hurdle is the removal of the meiotic spindle from MII oocytes. Traditional aspiration utilizes micromanipulation in conjunction with Hoechst staining and UV visualization to confirm the complete removal of spindle [13]. This method usually results in removal of a proportion of cytoplasm and potentially harmful UV irradiation. Recently, successful use of POLSCOPE to remove minimal cytoplasm along with the spindle was reported in nonhuman primates [15], which avoids the use of chemical stains like the Hoechst dye and UV irradiation of the oocytes. Table 1 shows a comparison of various publications on human SCNT; techniques used by various investigators and their success. Possibly the use of a hypoxic environment (6% oxygen) during embryo culture may have influenced the development of five blastocysts in the recently published study [13].

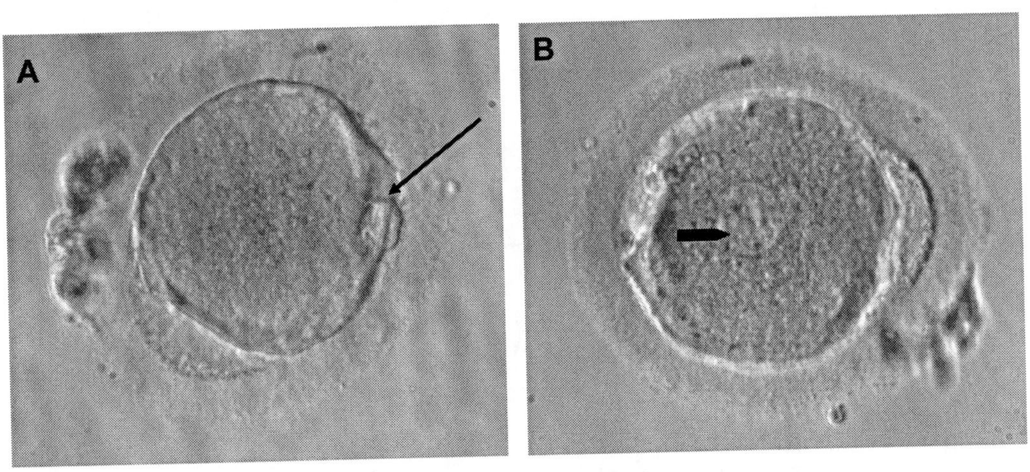

Figure 3. Pronuclei formation post parthenogenetic activation. Mature MII oocyte with the first polar body (arrow, A). Chemical activation initiates calcium flux, suppresses protein synthesis and induces pronuclei formation (block arrow, B) without completion of meiosis. Instead of releasing second polar body, the diploid activated MII oocyte enters mitosis and undergoes further cleavage.

Table 1. A Comparative Analysis of Technical Steps carried out by Various Investigators during Human SCNT

Se No	Reference	Eggs used for the study	Enucleation method	Somatic cell used for SCNT	Method of inserting somatic cell	Time post reconstruction prior to activation	Activation of egg post reconstruction	Culture medium & culture conditions	Success achieved
1	Cibelli et al, 2001	n= 71 Egg donors were women with one child	Piezo Electric Device to remove spindle	Adult skin fibroblast from skin biopsy	Piezo driven needle to inject somatic cell into egg cytoplasm	1- 3 hrs	5 uM calcium ionomycin for 4 min 2 mM DMAP for 3 hours	Commercial human IVF medium 37° C, 5% CO_2	6 cell stage embryo
2	Lavoir et al, 2005	Failed fertilized eggs n=51	Spindle was squeezed/ sucked out through a hole made in oocyte zona pellucida	CRL 7895 and BJ5 fibroblasts Serum starved	Piezo impact drive used to inject fibroblast into the egg cytoplasm	2- 3 hrs	AC & DC Electric Pulse used to activate the egg DMAP treatment not given	Co-cultured with BRL cells in KSOM medium 37° C, 5% CO_2	2 formed 3- 4 cell embryo
3	Stojkovic et al, 2005	Failed fertilized eggs, Good quality eggs n=36	Spindle extrusion by squeezing Hoechst stain used to visualize the spindle	Human Embryonic Stem cells Serum Starved	Somatic cell deposited in perivitelline space & electrofused with the egg cytoplast	2 hrs	10 uM Calcium Ionophore 5 min 2 mM DMAP for 4 hours	Commercial human IVF medium 37° C, 5% CO_2	One blastocyst but did not attach on feeder layer DNA fingerprinting comparison revealed successful SCNT

Table 1 (Continued)

Se No	Reference	Eggs used for the study	Enucleation method	Somatic cell used for SCNT	Method of inserting somatic cell	Time post reconstruction prior to activation	Activation of egg post reconstruction	Culture medium & culture conditions	Success achieved
4	Heindryckx et al, 2007	IVM GV eggs (n=61) Good MII eggs (n=54) Failed Fertilized (n=45) eggs	Removal of spindle through partially dissected zona Hoechst staining and UV exposure	Cumulus cells	Conventional ICSI method	2 hrs	10 uM calcium ionophore for 7 minutes (repeated after 30 minutes) 2 mM DMAP for 3 hours	Commercial human IVF medium 37° C, 5% CO2	Morula stage embryo obtained
5	French et al, 2008	Excess to reproductive need, good quality eggs n= 29	Extrusion/ Aspiration Hoechst staining done	Adult skin fibroblasts	Somatic cell deposited in perivitelline space & electrofused with the egg cytoplast	2 hrs	10 uM Calcium ionophore for 4 min 2 mM DMAP for 3 hours or 10 ug/ml cycloheximide & 2.5 ug/ml cytochalasin D	Commercial human IVF medium 37° C 5% CO2, 6% O2, 89% N2	5 SCNT blastocyst obtained Only one of these had donor cell genomic DNA and oocyte mtDNA
6	Present study	Good quality MII eggs from donors n= 15	Micromanipulator assisted aspiration under POLSCOPE	Fetal fibroblasts Serum starved	Conventional ICSI method	15 mins	5 uM Calcium Ionomycin for 5-10 mins 2 mM DMAP for 3 hours	Commercial human IVF medium 37° C 5% CO2, 6% O2, 89% N2	8- 10 cell embryo

The present study refined techniques for both spindle extraction and somatic cell insertion in the cytoplast, however due to the limited number of oocytes used for the study and the relatively short time allowed post - reconstruction for reprogramming of the donor nucleus by the cytoplast, may be the major factors for the limited development of the SCNT embryos produced. SCNT technology development is a steep learning curve for various researchers and further optimization is required prior to its clinical exploitation.

Failure to attach to the feeder layer and further proliferation by the parthenote morula (Figure 4D) was a setback to the study. However, it could possibly be because it was left in cleavage medium for almost forty-eight hours with the hope it may progress to blastocyst. Thereafter it was placed on feeder, but probably forty-eight hours of growth arrest was deleterious to the morula. In fact, recent literature provides evidence that we need not focus on obtaining SCNT or parthenote blastocyst, rather autologous cell lines could be derived from single blastomeres of early stage cleavage embryos [16]. Use of ACTH in place of FCS resulted in the derivation of mouse ES cell lines from single blastomeres with a high success rate [17].

If the process of SCNT has to provide clinical utility for cell therapy, success rate to derive SCNT embryonic stem cell lines need to be significantly improved. Instead of reprogramming a sperm nucleus, during SCNT, the egg cytoplasm has to reprogram a somatic cell. Wakayama [18] has discussed various factors that may help improve efficiency of the process. It is well documented that factors like the nature of activation method, timing of spindle removal, type of cytokinesis inhibitors used, addition of supplementary oocytes cytoplasm prior to SCNT, age and sex of donor or phase of donor cell cycle has little or no effect on overall efficiency of SCNT. However, a 5 fold- increase in success rate of mouse cloning from cumulus cells was observed by treating with Trichostatin A for 10 hours following oocytes activation. Thus it becomes evident that research efforts need to be focused on the basic understanding of nuclear reprogramming that take place when a somatic cell is introduced into an enucleated egg. The yet unidentified factors present in MII oocytes, which bring about DNA methylation and histone modification needs to be identified. A comparison of proteome and genome content of mature versus immature human eggs may provide valuable insights in this regard.

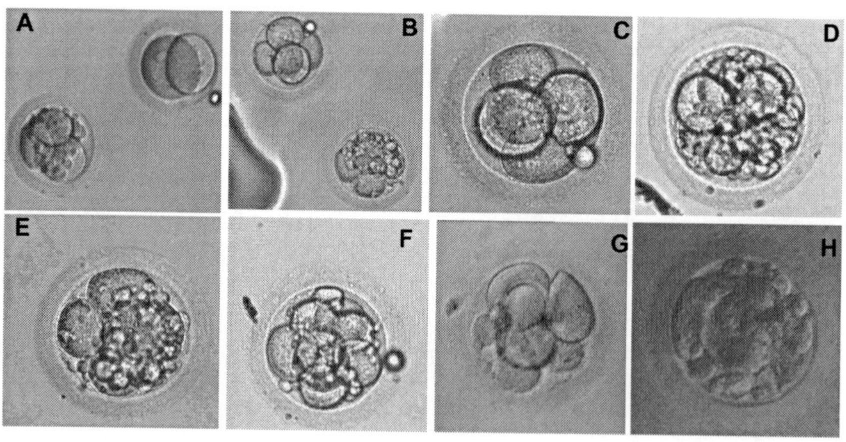

Figure 4. Embryo cleavage post activation after two (A), three (B- D) and four (E & F) days *in vitro;* another parthenote went up to compaction (G & H).

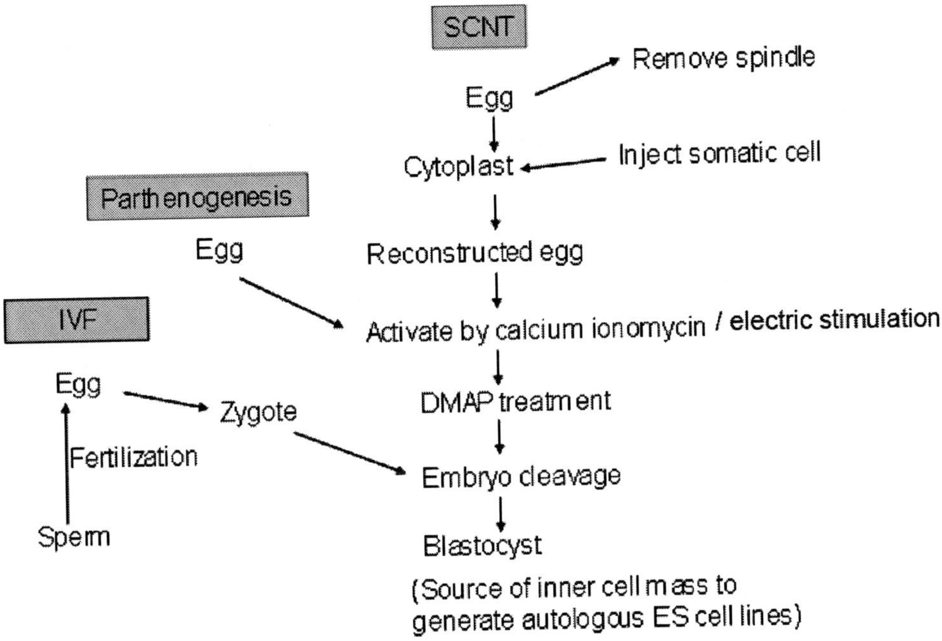

Figure 5. Technical relation between the process of IVF, Parthenogenesis and SCNT.

The three processes of IVF, SCNT and parthenogenesis are technically linked to each other (Figure 4). The prerequisites for effective SCNT studies are a functional IVF lab with efficient activation and embryo culture expertise. Proper infrastructures, dedicated incubators for SCNT embryo culture – separate from the ones which are frequently opened during micromanipulations, appropriate temperature and pH control during reconstruction of eggs are critical aspects that need to be kept in mind to achieve success following SCNT, in a manner similar to any standard ART facility.

Another question posed is: What are the culture media requirements for reconstructed eggs? Is it same as for IVF embryos or different? In the present study, the same embryo culture conditions and medium were used as for IVF embryos. Time interval post reconstruction, prior to activation is another crucial factor which needs to be determined.

Following the encouraging results obtained from these preliminary studies, a project to develop autologous embryonic stem cell lines by SCNT and parthenogenesis has been proposed to the Institute Ethics Committee of NIRRH and will subsequently be submitted to the National Apex Committee of Indian Council of Medical Research and Department of Biotechnology, Government of India for sanction. In India egg donors are regularly recruited in IVF clinics to help couples with female factor infertility. Excess oocytes from this egg donation program as well as from couples having eggs exceeding their reproductive needs will be sought for this research. Oocytes will be obtained after getting written informed consent of the couples. The researchers shall get oocytes without direct linkage information and will be unaware of the identity of the oocyte donor. However, detailed records will be maintained for each gamete, somatic cell or product of SCNT and parthenogenetically created embryo. This record will be sufficient to track back the SCNT or parthenogenetically embryo to the egg donor should the need arise.

Through this preliminary study we have gained a greater understanding of the logistics, process and technology involved in generating autologous ES cell lines. And although we were not successful in obtaining SCNT or parthenogenetic blastocysts, we feel India is poised to undertake such studies in near future.

Acknowledgments

The authors sincerely thank Union Minister for Health and Family Welfare, Government of India, Dr Ambumani Ramadoss; Dr NK Ganguly, former Director General, Indian Council for Medical Research, New Delhi; Dr MK Bhan, Secretary, Department of Biotechnology, New Delhi, Dr Chander Puri, former Director, NIRRH and Professors B. Williams and M. Holland, Monash Institute of Medical Research, Australia for encouragement and support. The Training Course to acquire SCNT technology was supported by Department of Biotechnology, Government of India, New Delhi, India.

References

[1] Mandal A, Tipnis S, Pal R, et al.: Characterization and *in vitro* differentiation potential of a new human embryonic stem cell line, Relicell hES1. *Differentiation.* 74,1-10 (2006).

[2] Inamdar M, Venu P, Ms S, et al.: Derivation and characterization of two sibling human embryonic stem cell lines from discarded Grade III embryos. *Stem Cells Dev.* (2008) Jul 10. [Epub ahead of print].

[3] Kumar N, Hinduja I, Nagvenkar P, et al.: Derivation and characterization of two genetically unique human embryonic stem cell lines on in-house-derived human feeders. *Stem Cells Dev.* (2008) Aug 12. [Epub ahead of print].

[4] Yamanaka S.: Induction of pluripotent stem cells from mouse fibroblasts by four transcription factors. *Cell Prolif.* 41, 51-6 (2008).

[5] Cibelli J : Is therapeutic cloning dead? *Science*; 318,1879- 80 (2007).

[6] Cervera RP, Stojkovic M: Somatic cell nuclear transfer- Progress and promise. *Stem Cells*. 26, 494- 495 (2008).

[7] Hall VJ, Stojkovic P and Stojkovic M.: Using therapeutic cloning to fight human disease: A conundrum or reality? *Stem Cells*. 30, 30 (2006).

[8] Cibelli JB, Kiessling AA, Cuniff K et al.: Somatic cell nuclear transfer in humans: pronuclear and early embryonic development. *J. Reg. Med.* 2, 25–31 (2001).

[9] Lu C, Lin G, Xie X et al.: Reconstruction of human embryos derived from somatic cells. *Chin. Science Bull.* 48, 1840–1843 (2003).

[10] Lavoir MC, Weier J, Conaghan J et al.: Poor development of human nuclear transfer embryos using failed fertilized oocytes. *Reprod. Biomed. Online*, 11, 740–744 (2005).

[11] Stojkovic M, Stojkovic P, Leary C et al.: Derivation of a human blastocyst after heterologous nuclear transfer to donated oocytes. *Reprod. Biomed. Online*.11, 226–231 (2005).

[12] Heindryckx B, De Sutter P, Gerris J et al.: Embryo development after successful somatic cell nuclear transfer to in vitro matured human germinal vesicle oocytes. *Hum. Reprod.* 22, 1982-1990 (2007).

[13] French AJ, Adams CA, Anderson LS et al.: Development of human cloned blastocysts following somatic cell nuclear transfer (SCNT) with adult fibroblasts. *Stem Cells.* 26, 485-493 (2008).

[14] Revazova ES, Turovets NA, Kochetkova OD et al.: Patient-specific stem cell lines derived from human parthenogenetic blastocysts. *Cloning and Stem Cells.* 9, 1- 18 (2007).

[15] Byrne JA, Pedersen DA, Clepper LL at al. Producing primate embryonic stem cells by somatic cell nuclear cell nuclear transfer. *Nature.*10, 1038 (2007).

[16] Klimanskaya I, Chung Y, Becker S, et al.: Derivation of human embryonic stem cells from single blastomeres. *Nat. Protoc.* 2, 1963-1972 (2007).

[17] Wakayama S, Hikichi T, Suetsugu R et al (2007) Efficient establishment of mouse embryonic stem cell lines from single blastomeres and polar bodies. *Stem Cells*, 25, 986- 993.

[18] Wakayama T.: Production of Cloned Mice and ES Cells from Adult Somatic Cells by Nuclear Transfer: How to Improve Cloning Efficiency?. *Reprod.. Dev.* 53, 13-26 (2007).*J.*

In: Stem Cell Therapy and Uses in Medical Treatment
Editor: Prasad S. Koka, pp. 93-104
ISBN: 978-1-61324-008-3

Chapter 6

Human Cord Blood Stem Cell Applications in Cell Therapy

Yu-Chen Gu, Mahendra S. Rao and Mohan C. Vemuri*
Stem Cells and Regenerative Medicine
Primary and Stem Cell Culture Systems
Life Technologies, 7335 Executive Way, Frederick, MD 21704, USA

Abstract

Human umbilical cord blood (UCB) is a valuable alternative source of ethically acceptable, clinically competent stem cells that is most likely closest to embryonic stem cells. Development of reliable methods for the expansion of cord blood stem cells is critical to ensure their clinical application. In the present article, advances in cord blood stem cell isolation, culture expansion methods through co-culture with human mesenchymal stem cells, culture optimization techniques with defined media and cord blood stem cell banking aspects have been reviewed. Refined methods of isolation as well as defined culture conditions of expansion that favor retention of stem cell phenotype and proper cryogenic storage can significantly increase the use of cord blood stem cells in human cell therapy applications.

Summary for Lay Readers

Following a baby's birth, the umbilical cord and placenta are usually discarded. However, recent scientific advances show that umbilical cord is a good source of stem cells. Stem cells are unspecialized cell types which can be differentiated into mature specific cell types that are found in tissues such as blood, heart, pancreas or muscle. Umbilical cord stem cells can be used like donated bone marrow cells to treat various

* Corresponding author: Mohan C. Vemuri, E-mail: Mohan.Vemuri@invitrogen.com; Phone: 240 379 4865; Fax: 240 379 4750

genetic diseases and cancers such as leukemia. Currently, more than 50 disorders can be treated with stem cells from the umbilical cord. In the present article, we have reviewed the process of stem cell isolation, cell culture expansion and stem cell banking aspects for the umbilical cord stem cells.

Keywords: hematopoietic stem cells; expansion; stem cell banking; self renewal; differentiation; cell therapy; umbilical cord blood.

Introduction

In broad terms, there are two types of stem cells, embryonic stem cells and adult stem cells. Embryonic stem cells (ESC) have great potential for cell therapy and can be noted from the first FDA approved clinical trials (www.washintonpost.com, Jan 23, 2009). But ESCs still retain their tendency to form tumors in animal transplant experiments which is a considerable concern. Besides, ESCs also have been associated with ethical controversy and issues about feeder cell free culture practices as well as the presence of animal derived products in the culture. Human umbilical cord blood (UCB) adult stem cells are closest in form and age to embryonic stem cells, and hence have high potential in regenerative medicine through cell therapy. Compared with peripheral blood stem cells and bone marrow stem cells, UCB stem cells have many advantages as an attractive stem cell source. Numerous studies feature the advantages of using UCB stem cell in cell therapy. First, UCB stem cells can be maintained and expanded in animal-free conditions and therefore the concerns over animal origin culture component are less. Second, UCB collection is non-invasive, safe and painless procedure to the mother and infant and the usage is not associated with ethical concerns. Third, the long term cell cryopreservation does not affect UCB stem cell proliferation and differentiation capacities [1]. Fourth, low incidence of graft versus host disease is noticed when UCB hematopoietic stem cell (HSC) is employed in transplantation compared with bone marrow HSC. Fifth, the yield of $CD34^+$ stem cells from UCB is higher than other sources, such as adult bone marrow [2]. Sixth, a higher degree tolerance for HLA-mismatches in recipients is noticed when UCB HSC is used compared with bone marrow from unrelated donor [3].

UCB HSCs have been used as a powerful tool for the treatment of several blood related diseases such as Fanconi anemia [4], leukemia [5], thalassemia, sickle cell disease [6]. Though the majority of recipients belong to the pediatric group, successful transplant in adults have also been reported. The Minnesota group [78], has pioneered double UCB grafts in order to overcome the cell dose limitation for larger patients. Recently Brunstein and colleagues published their experience in nearly 200 double UCB transplantation in both myeloablative and non-myeloablative regimen. They found double UCB transplantation is technically feasible, clinically safe, and increase eligibility of adult patients for transplantation [9].

UCB stem cells are likely the best alternative to ES cells as they can be used to derive tissues from different germ lineages. Except HSC, other types of stem cells are also found in UCB, such as dendritic stem cells [10], hepatocyte progenitor cells and pancreatic islet cells [11], and mesenchymal stem cells [12]. Major limitations in clinical use of cord blood HSC involve a) isolation of stem cells that are few in numbers and b) following their isolation, lack of appropriate cell culture expansion methods that allow these stem cells to grow without losing their stem cell phenotype. Current methods of isolation and expansion of stem cells from umbilical cord blood, the process of stem cell banking, and the ethical issues surrounding stem cell banking are reviewed in this article. The readers are directed to a review that has emphasized the implications of cord blood transplantation, HLA matching and future uses of cord blood [13].

Isolation of HSC from Human Cord Blood

The process of HSC isolation from cord blood begins with paperwork. Informed consent from the parents and Institutional Review Board approval (for studies to be performed) must be obtained prior to collection. Using strict aseptic techniques the cord blood is collected after the umbilical cord has been cut and either *in vivo* after the baby is born, before the expulsion of the placenta, or *in vitro* after the placenta is delivered [14]. *In vitro* collection of cord blood is performed by placing the delivered placenta in a specialized funnel-like holding apparatus. Trained personnel collect the blood intravenously into the anticoagulant-containing collection bag by a gravitational flow using sterile technique. In either of the collection methods, the cord blood is collected in special bag containing citrate phosphate dextrose adenine (CPDA), CPD, acid citrate dextrose (ACD) or heparin as an anticoagulant [15]; [16]. During the collection the blood bag was shaken gently, so that the anticoagulant freely mixed with UCB. A new two-step collection procedure has shown to produce significantly higher concentrations of cells. After normal collection, additional cells are harvested from the placenta by flowing 50mL of "heparinized saline" through the placenta. This additional step adds approximately 15% more nucleated cells to the sample, which could allow samples to be utilized in larger patients [17].

In an effort to enrich HSC population, red blood cells (RBC) are removed (called RBC depletion) using the Ficoll-Hypaque density gradient separation technique. In this procedure, each cord blood sample is layered on top of Ficoll (polygeline or gelatin can also be used in modified methods) and centrifuged to separate the cells by density. The denser red blood cells will collect at the bottom, and the stem cells can be harvested at inter-phase along with other mononuclear cells. In an alternate method, hydroxyethylstarch (HES) is mixed with the cord blood sample and centrifuged at low speed [18]. There are two fractions that result from this centrifugation: white blood cell (WBC)-rich plasma and WBC-poor plasma. The WBC-poor plasma is discarded, and the WBC-rich fraction is re-centrifuged at a higher speed. Following this second centrifugation, the supernatant is discarded. In addition, ammonium sulfate or other red blood cell lysis solutions (Becton Dickinson FACS Lysing Solution) can be used to deplete RBCs, and the post-lysed cell fraction is collected.

Post RBC depletion, a small portion of sample was taken for cellular composition analysis. The rest are prepared for storage by adding 10% DMSO containing Dextran 40. Samples are then cooled in a temperature controlled freezer at 1°C per minute until the sample reaches -100°C, and placed in liquid nitrogen for long term storage [19]. Results of samples tested prior to cryopreservation can be used to estimate the probability of success for transplantation. Cells are tested for total nucleated cell count using a hemocytometer. Flow cytometry and fluorescence activated cell sorting (FACS) analysis are performed to determine the number of $CD34^+$ cells. In general, samples with higher numbers of $CD34^+$ cells have an increased probability of successful transplantation [20] in which the criteria for selecting cord blood samples is based primarily on the number of $CD34^+$ cells. A recent study on unrelated UCB stem cell transplant in total of 102 patients showed CD34 cell dose was the one factor consistently identified as significantly associated with rate of engraftment, treatment related mortality and survival. There is a high probability of survival in recipients of UCB grafts that are disparate in no more than two human leukocyte antigens when the grafts contain at least 1.7×10^5 $CD34^+$ cells per kilogram of recipient's body weight [21].

Upon completion of the $CD34^+$ cell counts, proliferative ability of HSC is determined by CFU assay. The cells are plated in semi-solid methylcellulose culture medium along with growth factors, the number of colonies formed after 14 days is used to calculate the number of colony-forming units (CFUs) [19]. All of these analytical tests are used to characterize each batch of HSCs in UCB samples.

Expansion of Human UCB Stem Cells

Expansion has been suggested as a means of obtaining larger cell numbers to improve outcomes in patients with higher body weight. Expansion should ideally lead to cell population, which would reduce long periods of neutropenia and thrombocy topenia associated with UCB transplants. The major challenge of stem cell expansion from any source, including UCB, is getting true undifferentiated HSCs to increase number in culture. The expansion of UCB HSC has been a major determinant for clinical use. Due to the fact that the number of HSCs within an UCB donation is low (approximately a few million) and typical clinical transplant treatments in adults require about 7 to 10 million total nucleated cells per kilogram of weight (NIH Stem Cell information page, Available at: http://stemcells.nih.gov/info/scireport/chapter4.asp.). Initial efforts to expand UCB stem cells *ex vivo* have resulted in expansion of mature rather than immature HSC [22]. Thus efforts to increase the number of HSC in *ex vivo* expansion are paramount. Culture systems relying on cytokines to support UCB HSC has limited success. The commonly used cytokines for expansion cultures include granulocyte colony stimulating factor, stem cell factor, thrombopoietin, granulocyte macrophage colony stimulating factor, interleukin 3 and 6, Flt-3 ligand. The majority studies in which UCB HSC are cultured in cytokine supplemented condition show that short term culture results in a moderate increase in SCID repopulating cells (SRC), but loss of SRC if the cultures are extended for longer than 9 days. In addition, cytokines driven HSC ex vivo culture require stroma for optimal maintenance of graft quality [23]; [24]; [25].

Some more recent data showed the improvement of *ex vivo* culture in different settings. For example, the Piacibello group reported a striking increase of SRC number of cord blood cells after 16 weeks of culture [26]. Summers and colleagues reported a very high incidence of long term culture initiating cell (LTC-IC) and colony forming cells (CFC) expansion in CD133+ cell culture [27]. Araki demonstrated that the treatment of cord blood $CD34^+$ cells with chromatin-modifying agents 5-aza-2'-deoxycytidine and trichostatin A resulted in almost 10 fold expansion of total SRC numbers after 9 days of culture [28]. Another research group led by Dr. Lodish developed a serum-free culture medium supplemented with IGF binding protein 2 (IGFBP2) and angiopoietin-like 5 protein, together with SCF, TPO and FGF-1 to culture and expand human UCB HSC.

This system supports an approximately 20 fold net expansion of repopulating HSCs [29]. A number of developmentally important, non-hematopoietic growth factors have also recently emerged to support HSC self-renewal during *ex vivo* expansion. These include sonic hedgehog [30], bone morphogenic protein [31], and fibroblast growth factor-1 [32]. A recent report suggested that valproic acid, a common medication used for treating seizure, enhanced UCB HSC $CD34^+$ cells and maintain their cell cycle progression [33]. In addition to HSC expansion in cytokine supplemented condition, co-culture of the cells on feeder cells, or a combination of both have also been used extensively.

Do Feeder Cells Enhance Cord Blood Stem Cell Expansion?

It has long been accepted that *in vivo* HSCs are found in close association with important cellular and extracellular components in discrete microenvironment. Several feeder cell types have been attempted to enhance expansion of cord blood stem cells. A few cell types which have been studied include stromal cells, umbilical vein endothelial cells, cord blood derived unrestricted somatic stem cells and bone-marrow mesenchymal stem cells. Culturing of cord blood stem cells on a feeder layer of human mesenchymal stem cells provides a superior culture environment to the culture supplemented only with cytokines [34]; [35] and resulted in 10- and 14-fold expansion of total nucleated cells (TNC) and $CD34^+$ cells [34].

Another feeder cell type is human umbilical vein endothelial cells (HUVEC). Cord blood cells grown in culture with HUVEC cells and supplemented with either 3 growth factors [Stem cell factor (SCF), vascular endothelial growth factor (VEGF) and interleukin-1 (IL-1)] or 5 growth factors [FMS-like tyrosine kinase 3- (FLT3 ligand), interleukin-6 (IL6), SCF, VEGF and IL-1] resulted in an expansion of total nucleated cells of 55- and 77-fold for 3 and 5 growth factors, respectively. In addition, the population of $CD34^+$ cells was increased by 15- and 23-fold for 3 and 5 growth factors, respectively. Interestingly, the HUVEC cells were primary cell lines, derived from the same umbilical cord as the donor cord blood cells [36].

The expansion profile of cord blood stem cells in these two experimental regimens is summarized in Table 1. As can be noticed in Table 1, feeder cells do provide a beneficial environment for the expansion of cord blood cells.

In conclusion, when cultured with feeder cells and cytokine supplements, the number of $CD34^+$ cells can be increased by approximately 15-fold. One factor in considering the choice of culture conditions for expanding cord blood stem cells is the ability to maintain the primitive stem cell types and prevent differentiation. Overall, the ability to retain and multiply more “primitive” cell types like “cobblestone area forming cells” seems to decrease as other cell types proliferate [34]. Although co-culture expansion system is not clinically useful for clinical CB *ex vivo* expansion, dissecting the feeder cell-HSC signaling events that contribute to the maintenance and expansion of HSC is an approach that may identify factors that can be translated into clinically relevant systems.

Table 1. Fold-increase of cord blood cells when grown with feeder cell types

Feeder Cell Type	Autologous HUVEC		Human Mesenchymal stem cells
Supplements	3 growth factors	5 growth factors	Cytokines
Total nucleated cells (TNC)	55 – fold	77 – fold	10 - fold
$CD34^+$ cells	15 - fold	23 - fold	14 - fold

Can Creative Cell Culture Systems Help Maintain Progenitor Cells?

Proliferation and differentiation of stem cells *in vivo* is controlled in part by signals from the extracellular matrix, cell-cell interactions and cell-matrix interactions (NIH Stem Cell information page, Available at: http://stemcells.nih.gov/info/scireport/chapter4.asp.). In research performed to gain a better understanding of the optimal cell culture conditions for controlling the stem cell expansion, various cell culture manipulation techniques were examined. In one recent study, the authors defined their culture manipulation as a "global culture manipulation (GCM) technique" [37]. Their technique included repeated selection of cells and media exchanges, where differentiating cells (lin^+) were removed from the culture. Measurements of HSCs grown in cytokine-supplemented culture showed that the number of cells which were differentiated (lin^+) increased as the length of culture increased. In addition, measurements of two typical negative regulators TGF-β1 and MIP-1α showed that their concentrations increased as the length of culture time increased. Parameters investigated were the removal of cells which had begun to differentiate (lin^+) and the effect of media exchanges on the final population of cells in culture at the completion of the experiment. A combination treatment of the cultured cells, where differentiated cells (lin^+) were removed and media was exchanged, seemed to have a preferential success in maintaining long-term culture initiating cell (LTC-IC) populations, as determined by LTC-IC assays [37].

The use of autologous feeder cells might be beneficial in ensuring that the cell therapy approaches can move forward to a clinical setting. Optimal cell culture conditions may vary depending on the purpose for expansion. However, results from experimentation proved that culture techniques are possible which will help select and maintain cells more "multipotent" in nature, as proven by both LTC-IC assays and *in vivo* studies in NOD/SCID mice [37]. These techniques, in combination with additional research into creating clinically safe immortal cell lines, may help scientists find the most robust and consistent methods to expand human UCB stem cells.

The Potential for Permanent Stem Cell Lines

Current research emphasis involves HSC and cord blood stem cell short-term expansion for immediate use in clinical transplantation. To meet the increasing needs of stem cells in sufficient numbers, establishing permanent cell lines might help scientists cope with the demand. In addition to the tendency to differentiate, another issue to overcome in the culture of adult stem cells is senescence. One method of overcoming senescence which would allow cells to divide nearly indefinitely is stabilizing the telomere length on chromosomes within the cells. The ability to bypass senescence was investigated through genetic manipulation of the hTERT (human Telomerase Reverse Transcriptase) gene (gene controlling expression of telomerase) as well as treatment with other factors to bypass cell division control [38]. In their studies, several experimental arms and combinations were tested such as genetic modification of the hTERT gene, introduction of human papillomavirus (HPV) type 16 and 17 E6 and E7 vectors, and combinations of both. Results showed that the combination treatment to express the hTERT gene along with treatment to express the HPV E6 and E7 genes proved to be successful. Cells were immortalized as well as genomically stable. In total, the researchers created a total of 11 cell lines – 9 of which were a result of the combination of the hTERT and HPV E6/E7 genes. It should be noted that the analysis of the cell lines was restricted to 5 lines – three of which were created from the hTERT + HPV E6/E7 treatment. Two of the cell lines created from the hTERT + HPV E6/E7 were tested in NOD/SCID mice and proven to be non-tumorigenic. However, when the same cell lines were transduced with oncogenes (v-H-*ras* or *BCR-ABL*) and tested in NOD/SCID mice, the cells were able to become tumorigenic. Therefore, gene manipulation approaches to enhance the number of stem cells in cord blood have to be more closely scrutinized and re-evaluated, before human use of such immortalized cell lines with HPV viruses.

Umbilical Cord Blood (UCB) Banking

The first UCB stem cell bank was established by Indiana University [13]. The blood stored through Indiana University's cord blood bank was used to treat a patient with Fanconi anemia [39]. The successful use of UCB on various clinical applications mobilized the various government agencies, such as the National Institute of Health, to begin awarding grants to UCB banks and research centers to study the quality and safe use of UCB stem cells for therapeutic purposes. Over 7000 UCB transplants have been performed worldwide. Successful UCB transplant programs led to the establishment of two types of UCB banks: public banks and for-profit private banks. Through July 2008, a total of 82 UCB units were released for clinical use. Among these, 57% UCB units have been used for traditional transplantation and the rest 43% have been used for regenerative medicine. The indication for regenerative medicine autologous infusions were cerebral palsy, brain injury, type 1 diabetes and a rare immune disorder (Weinthal J ASH abstract, 2008).

Cord blood banks may vary based on the type of blood donation. Allogenic donations are donations that are made for use in other individuals and are mostly associated with public banks. The first public cord blood banking of unrelated umbilical cord blood began in New York in 1993, soon after similar banks were established around the world, including Paris, Milan and Sydney. A well match donor is pivotal to the success of allogenic transplant. The inheritance of the human leukocyte antigen (HLA) means that there is only 25% chance a sibling will have a full match. About 70% of patients do not have a suitable donor in their family and an unrelated donor stem cell source must be found. Due to the fact that UCB is more permissive of donor-host tissue mismatch, it allows a greater number of patients to benefit from a smaller donor pool. Public cord blood banks were established essentially to overcome this problem for majority of allogenic transplant patients. Autologous donations are donations of cord blood for use in the child that it originated from in the event that it is needed for treatment later in life [13]. Some private banks also accept allogenic donations intended for use in immediate family members. UCB collected from the general public is similar to normal blood donation for public banks, but private banks usually collect and ship to its destination with a particular cost associated with it. When the stem cells are stored for public use, there are certain standards and criteria that the blood must meet before the blood is deemed available for storage and transplantation. Rigorous screening includes testing for infectious disease, red blood cell count, Human Leukocyte Antigen (HLA) and cell count evaluation [40]. Samples failing to meet these criteria are not stored in any bank and are virtually useless. However, the rigorous testing on UCB samples in private banks is limited because it is used for autologous donations.

A number of for profit private banking are available that encourage parents to bank their infants' cord blood as a form of "biological insurance." The cost of private banks' enrollment and collection fees vary from about \$600 to \$1,900, with annual storage costs ranging from about \$85 to \$125. However, many private banks also offer free or discounted banking if a sibling or family member has a medical condition that makes him a candidate now, or in the future, for a cord blood transplant. Currently, there is no direct and clear evidence of the safety and effectiveness of autologous cord blood stem cell transplantation for the treatment of malignancies. The potential for children needing their own cord blood stem cells for future autologous use is controversial. The range of the likelihood estimates is from 1 in 1000 to more than 1 in 200,000 [41]. The third type of cord blood bank is a directed donation. Directed donations are free of cost and can be used for immediate family members known to have an illness [13]. There are many factors to consider when collecting cord blood cells to determine their potential viability for therapeutic purposes. Quality of cord blood samples can be determined by a number of factors such as high levels of nucleated $CD34^+$ cell counts as in first born infants, increased birth weight, prolonged labor and pregnancies that are more than 34 weeks gestation [42][43][44].

Regulation of cord blood banking is a recent phenomenon. Regulation is critical because cord blood for use in an allogeneic nature must meet specific criteria. If these specifications are not met, individuals using donated cord blood could become infected with diseases such as HIV, defeating the purpose of cord blood for treatment. In recent years, the Food and Drug Administration (FDA) proposed regulations and required all cord blood banks to register with them [13]. Quality assurance violations at cord blood banks could potentially result in fines or closures, much like consequences of violations imposed on organizations within the pharmaceutical industry. It is important that the umbilical cord banking industry is regulated to ensure the safety of the public. In addition, a significant education campaign by government agencies and the medical community should be conducted to ensure that the average person understands the pros and cons of the research. Regulation of stem cell banks, education for the public and continued research to improve the procedures involved in cord blood stem cell research will be the key to the success of these cells for therapeutic purposes.

Conclusion

Technology for the isolation, expansion, cryopreservation and utilization of cord blood stem cells continues to evolve. Cord blood stem cells, in large enough quantities, may eventually replace the use of hematopoietic stem cells isolated from bone marrow. This is a major benefit to patients and bone marrow donors alike, eliminating the pain associated with the donation process. Because the donation of cord blood stem cells is virtually non-intrusive, the number of donations may increase significantly. The cord blood cells, because they are less differentiated, allow for a greater difference in the HLA-type between recipients and donors without the risk of rejection. Techniques for isolating stem cells from UCB have been well defined. Advancements in the expansion of cord blood stem cells continue to occur and improve both the cell number achieved as well as the ability to isolate the most primitive stem cells available. The quality of cord blood banking is critical to the success of using cord blood treatments as routine clinical practice. Future research for successful utilization of UCB stem cells in transplantation depends on the advances made in key areas primarily comprising but not exclusively limited to 1. Ex vivo expansion potential with clinical-grade cytokine cocktails 2. Engraftment ability of UCB stem cells following ex vivo expansion 2. Multi-cord transplant possibility 3. Use of Mesenchymal stem cells as co-transplant cells to facilitate engraftment 4. UCB stem cell dose required for adult patients 5. Conditioning regimen with UCB stem cells and GVHD prophylaxis. Further research will help ensure that cord blood stem cells can be used in the treatment of a wide variety of diseases and is available to large patient populations.

References

[1] Broxmeyer, HE; Srour, EF; Hangoc, G; Cooper, S; Anderson, SA; Bodine, DM. High-efficiency recovery of functional hematopoietic progenitor and stem cells from human cord blood cryopreserved for 15 years. *Proc. Natl. Acad. Sci. USA*. 2003, 100(2), 645-50.

[2] Hows, JM; Marsh, JC; Bradley, BA; Luft, T; Coutinho, L; Testa, NG; Dexter, TM. Human cord blood: a source of transplantable stem cells? *Bone Marrow Transplant*. 1992, 9 Suppl 1, 105-8.

[3] Rubinstein, P. Placental blood-derived hematopoietic stem cells for unrelated bone marrow reconstitution. *J Hematother*. 1993, 2(2), 207-10.

[4] de Medeiros, CR; Silva, LM; Pasquini, R. Unrelated cord blood transplantation in a Fanconi anemia patient using fludarabine-based conditioning. *Bone Marrow Transplant*. 2001, 28(1), 110-2.

[5] Jacobsohn, DA; Hewlett, B; Ranalli, M; Seshadri, R; Duerst, R; Kletzel, M. Outcomes of unrelated cord blood transplants and allogeneic-related hematopoietic stem cell transplants in children with high-risk acute lymphocytic leukemia. *Bone Marrow Transplant*. 2004, 34(10), 901-7.

[6] Locatelli, F; Rocha, V; Reed, W; Bernaudin, F; Ertem, M; Grafakos, S; Brichard, B; Li, X; Nagler, A; Giorgiani, G; Haut, PR; Brochstein, JA; Nugent, DJ; Blatt, J; Woodard, P; Kurtzberg, J; Rubin, CM; Miniero, R; Lutz, P; Raja, T; Roberts, I; Will, AM; Yaniv,

I; Vermylen, C; Tannoia, N; Garnier, F; Ionescu, I; Walters, MC; Lubin, BH; Gluckman, E. Related umbilical cord blood transplantation in patients with thalassemia and sickle cell disease. *Blood*. 2003, 101(6), 2137-43.

[7] Barker, JN; Weisdorf, DJ; DeFor, TE; Blazar, BR; McGlave, PB; Miller, JS; Verfaillie, CM; Wagner, JE. Transplantation of 2 partially HLA-matched umbilical cord blood units to enhance engraftment in adults with hematologic malignancy. *Blood*. 2005, 105(3), 1343-7.

[8] Barker, JN; Weisdorf, DJ; Wagner, JE. Creation of a double chimera after the transplantation of umbilical-cord blood from two partially matched unrelated donors. *N Engl. J. Med*. 2001, 344(24), 1870-1.

[9] Brunstein, CG; Baker, KS; Wagner, JE. Umbilical cord blood transplantation for myeloid malignancies. *Curr. Opin. Hematol*. 2007, 14(2), 162-9.

[10] Guo, G; Chen, S; Zhang, J; Luo, L; Yu, J; Dong, H; Xu, H; Su, Z; Wu, L. Antitumor activity of a fusion of esophageal carcinoma cells with dendritic cells derived from cord blood. *Vaccine*. 2005, 23(45), 5225-30.

[11] McGuckin, CP; Forraz, N; Baradez, MO; Navran, S; Zhao, J; Urban, R; Tilton, R; Denner, L. Production of stem cells with embryonic characteristics from human umbilical cord blood. *Cell Prolif*. 2005, 38(4), 245-55.

[12] Hutson, EL; Boyer, S; Genever, PG. Rapid isolation, expansion, and differentiation of osteoprogenitors from full-term umbilical cord blood. *Tissue Eng*. 2005, 11(9-10), 1407-20.

[13] Moise, KJ, Jr. Umbilical cord stem cells. *Obstet Gynecol*. 2005, 106(6), 1393-407.

[14] Bradley, MB; Cairo, MS. Cord blood immunology and stem cell transplantation. *Hum. Immunol*. 2005, 66(5), 431-46.

[15] Rubinstein, P; Dobrila, L; Rosenfield, RE; Adamson, JW; Migliaccio, G; Migliaccio, AR; Taylor, PE; Stevens, CE. Processing and cryopreservation of placental/umbilical cord blood for unrelated bone marrow reconstitution. *Proc. Natl. Acad. Sci USA*. 1995, 92(22), 10119-22.

[16] Broxmeyer, HE; Douglas, GW; Hangoc, G; Cooper, S; Bard, J; English, D; Arny, M; Thomas, L; Boyse, EA. Human umbilical cord blood as a potential source of transplantable hematopoietic stem/progenitor cells. *Proc. Natl. Acad. Sci. USA*. 1989, 86(10), 3828-32.

[17] Bornstein, R; Flores, AI; Montalban, MA; del Rey, MJ; de la Serna, J; Gilsanz, F. A modified cord blood collection method achieves sufficient cell levels for transplantation in most adult patients. *Stem Cells*. 2005, 23(3), 324-34.

[18] Laroche, V; McKenna, DH; Moroff, G; Schierman, T; Kadidlo, D; McCullough, J. Cell loss and recovery in umbilical cord blood processing: a comparison of postthaw and postwash samples. *Transfusion*. 2005, 45(12), 1909-16.

[19] Hubel, A; Carlquist, D; Clay, M; McCullough, J. Liquid storage, shipment, and cryopreservation of cord blood. *Transfusion*. 2004, 44(4), 518-25.

[20] Van Haute, I; Lootens, N; De Buck, K; Verdegen, L; Vander Steene, V; Desmet, S; Craeye, D; Vandekerckhove, B. Selecting cord blood units for storage by $CD34^+$ cell counts. *Transfusion*. 2005, 45(3), 455-7.

[21] Wagner, JE; Barker, JN; DeFor, TE; Baker, KS; Blazar, BR; Eide, C; Goldman, A; Kersey, J; Krivit, W; MacMillan, ML; Orchard, PJ; Peters, C; Weisdorf, DJ; Ramsay, NK; Davies, SM. Transplantation of unrelated donor umbilical cord blood in 102

patients with malignant and nonmalignant diseases: influence of CD34 cell dose and HLA disparity on treatment-related mortality and survival. *Blood*. 2002, 100(5), 1611-8.

[22] Rice, A; Flemming, C; Case, J; Stevenson, J; Gaudry, L; Vowels, M. Comparative study of the in vitro behavior of cord blood subpopulations after short-term cytokine exposure. *Bone Marrow Transplant*. 1999, 23(3), 211-20.

[23] Bhatia, M; Bonnet, D; Kapp, U; Wang, JC; Murdoch, B; Dick, JE. Quantitative analysis reveals expansion of human hematopoietic repopulating cells after short-term ex vivo culture. *J. Exp. Med*. 1997, 186(4), 619-24.

[24] Wineman, J; Moore, K; Lemischka, I; Muller-Sieburg, C. Functional heterogeneity of the hematopoietic microenvironment: rare stromal elements maintain long-term repopulating stem cells. *Blood*. 1996, 87(10), 4082-90.

[25] Breems, DA; Blokland, EA; Siebel, KE; Mayen, AE; Engels, LJ; Ploemacher, RE. Stroma-contact prevents loss of hematopoietic stem cell quality during ex vivo expansion of $CD34^+$ mobilized peripheral blood stem cells. *Blood*. 1998, 91(1), 111-7.

[26] Gammaitoni, L; Weisel, KC; Gunetti, M; Wu, KD; Bruno, S; Pinelli, S; Bonati, A; Aglietta, M; Moore, MA; Piacibello, W. Elevated telomerase activity and minimal telomere loss in cord blood long-term cultures with extensive stem cell replication. *Blood*. 2004, 103(12), 4440-8.

[27] Summers, YJ; Heyworth, CM; de Wynter, EA; Hart, CA; Chang, J; Testa, NG. AC133+ G0 cells from cord blood show a high incidence of long-term culture-initiating cells and a capacity for more than 100 million-fold amplification of colony-forming cells in vitro. *Stem Cells*. 2004, 22(5), 704-15.

[28] Araki, H; Mahmud, N; Milhem, M; Nunez, R; Xu, M; Beam, CA; Hoffman, R. Expansion of human umbilical cord blood SCID-repopulating cells using chromatin-modifying agents. *Exp. Hematol*. 2006, 34(2), 140-9.

[29] Zhang, CC; Kaba, M; Iizuka, S; Huynh, H; Lodish, HF. Angiopoietin-like 5 and IGFBP2 stimulate ex vivo expansion of human cord blood hematopoietic stem cells as assayed by NOD/SCID transplantation. *Blood*. 2008, 111(7), 3415-23.

[30] Bhardwaj, G; Murdoch, B; Wu, D; Baker, DP; Williams, KP; Chadwick, K; Ling, LE; Karanu, FN; Bhatia, M. Sonic hedgehog induces the proliferation of primitive human hematopoietic cells via BMP regulation. *Nat Immunol*. 2001, 2(2), 172-80.

[31] Bhatia, M; Bonnet, D; Wu, D; Murdoch, B; Wrana, J; Gallacher, L; Dick, JE. Bone morphogenetic proteins regulate the developmental program of human hematopoietic stem cells. *J. Exp. Med*. 1999, 189(7), 1139-48.

[32] de Haan, G; Weersing, E; Dontje, B; van Os, R; Bystrykh, LV; Vellenga, E; Miller, G. In vitro generation of long-term repopulating hematopoietic stem cells by fibroblast growth factor-1. *Dev. Cell*. 2003, 4(2), 241-51.

[33] Seet, LF; Teng, E; Lai, YS; Laning, J; Kraus, M; Wnendt, S; Merchav, S; Chan, SL. Valproic acid enhances the engraftability of human umbilical cord blood hematopoietic stem cells expanded under serum-free conditions. *Eur. J. Haematol*. 2009, 82(2), 124-32.

[34] Robinson, SN; Ng, J; Niu, T; Yang, H; McMannis, JD; Karandish, S; Kaur, I; Fu, P; Del Angel, M; Messinger, R; Flagge, F; de Lima, M; Decker, W; Xing, D; Champlin, R; Shpall, EJ. Superior ex vivo cord blood expansion following co-culture with bone

marrow-derived mesenchymal stem cells. *Bone Marrow Transplant.* 2006, 37(4), 359-66.

[35] Jang, YK; Jung, DH; Jung, MH; Kim, DH; Yoo, KH; Sung, KW; Koo, HH; Oh, W; Yang, YS; Yang, SE. Mesenchymal stem cells feeder layer from human umbilical cord blood for ex vivo expanded growth and proliferation of hematopoietic progenitor cells. *Ann. Hematol.* 2006, 85(4), 212-25.

[36] Yildirim, S; Boehmler, AM; Kanz, L; Mohle, R. Expansion of cord blood $CD34^+$ hematopoietic progenitor cells in coculture with autologous umbilical vein endothelial cells (HUVEC) is superior to cytokine-supplemented liquid culture. *Bone Marrow Transplant.* 2005, 36(1), 71-9.

[37] Madlambayan, GJ; Rogers, I; Kirouac, DC; Yamanaka, N; Mazurier, F; Doedens, M; Casper, RF; Dick, JE; Zandstra, PW. Dynamic changes in cellular and microenvironmental composition can be controlled to elicit in vitro human hematopoietic stem cell expansion. *Exp. Hematol.* 2005, 33(10), 1229-39.

[38] Akimov, SS; Ramezani, A; Hawley, TS; Hawley, RG. Bypass of senescence, immortalization, and transformation of human hematopoietic progenitor cells. *Stem Cells.* 2005, 23(9), 1423-33.

[39] Gluckman, E; Broxmeyer, HA; Auerbach, AD; Friedman, HS; Douglas, GW; Devergie, A; Esperou, H; Thierry, D; Socie, G; Lehn, P; et al. Hematopoietic reconstitution in a patient with Fanconi's anemia by means of umbilical-cord blood from an HLA-identical sibling. *N. Engl. J. Med.* 1989, 321(17), 1174-8.

[40] Gunning, J. Umbilical cord cell banking--implications for the future. *Toxicol. Appl. Pharmacol.* 2005, 207(2 Suppl), 538-43.

[41] Johnson, FL. Placental blood transplantation and autologous banking--caveat emptor. *J. Pediatr. Hematol Oncol.* 1997, 19(3), 183-6.

[42] Brunstein, CG; Wagner, JE. Umbilical cord blood transplantation and banking. *Annu. Rev. Med.* 2006, 57, 403-17.

[43] Fasouliotis, SJ; Schenker, JG. Human umbilical cord blood banking and transplantation: a state of the art. *Eur. J. Obstet Gynecol. Reprod Biol.* 2000, 90(1), 13-25.

[44] Kurtzberg, J; Cairo, MS; Fraser, JK; Baxter-Lowe, L; Cohen, G; Carter, SL; Kernan, NA. Results of the cord blood transplantation (COBLT) study unrelated donor banking program. *Transfusion.* 2005, 45(6), 842-55.

In: Stem Cell Therapy and Uses in Medical Treatment
Editor: Prasad S. Koka, pp. 105-115
ISBN: 978-1-61324-008-3

Chapter 7

Cancer Stem Cells: An Approach to Identify Newer Therapeutic Targets

Sweta Srivastava* and Sudhir Krishna
National Centre for Biological Sciences, TIFR, Bangalore, India

Abstract

Several studies have shown the existence of cancer stem cells and suggested that they might have a role to play in chemotherapy resistance and radioresistance. Their survival skills may be the contributing factor to incomplete remission of tumors and relapse of tumors periodically followed with metastasis. The irrefutable proof of existence of cancer stem cells in hematopoietic system made way for studies with solid tumors in quest for a similar phenomenon which may be exploited to tumor therapy. Advances have been made in this field and one is poised to utilize properties of the cancer stem cells to generate fresh drugs. Recent finding suggesting ROS related genes as one of the mechanisms by which the cancer stem cells can generate resistance is a hope towards new therapeutic avenues.

Introduction

The cancer stem cell hypothesis has two arguments. First being the cellular origin of tumors, including the argument that tumors arise from tissue stem cells. The second hypothesis being the tumor is driven by a population that has "stem cell properties." Analysis of tumorigenic properties of the cells of a tumor suggests that not all the cells from a tumor

---

* Corresponding Author: Sweta Srivastava, Address: National Centre for Biological Sciences, TIFR, UAS-GKVK Campus, Bangalore 560065, India. Telephone: +918023666071; Fax: +918023636662; Email ID: sweta@ncbs.res.in

have the potential to generate new tumor upon transplantation. There is a complex heterogeneity in the tumors. Not only amongst the tumor subtypes but heterogeneity is also observed within a tumor population, with cell having distinct properties with respect to proliferation and differentiation. Cancer stem cells represent one such population in the tumor. The concept that tumors contain cell populations with stem cell properties was also suggested by in vitro "clonogenic assays" that showed subpopulations of tumor cells with increased proliferative capacity. The evidence of existence of this pool of cells first surfaced from studies by Bonnet and Dick [1]. They suggested that there is a relatively small population (0.01-1%) of cell that has enhanced tumorgenic property. They showed that only $CD34^{+}/CD38^{-}$ cells purified from patients with acute myeloid leukemia were able to generate tumors in NOD/SCID mice, which were histologically similar to the donor. Since then one has seen the characterization of this population in various other tumors including Brain [2], Breast [3], Colon [4], Ovary [5], Pancreas [6] and Prostate [7, 8]. This tumor subset, that has ability to self-renew and generate diverse cells that form tumor, is referred to as the cancer stem cell (CSC). These cells were termed cancer stem cells as they phenocopied stem-like properties, sustained continual proliferation, exist in tumors as a distinct population, which may cause relapse and metastasis. Therefore, development of specific therapies targeted at CSCs holds hope for improvement of survival and quality of life of cancer patients, especially for sufferers of metastatic disease. There is an ensuing debate on the cell of origin of these CSCs - whether they arise from stem cells (with genetic alterations) or from a differentiated population of progenitor cells that have acquired abilities to self-renew. There are evidences which support the notion that self-renewal can be activated in progenitors thereby transforming them into cancers. An example includes, MLL-AF9 activates self renewal in granulocyte-macrophage progenitor resultantly forming leukemic stem cells [9].

Isolation of Cancer Stem Cells

The cancer stem cell hypothesis has gained impetus recently due to advances in stem cell biology and successful development of new animal models to measure self-renewal. The serial transplantation of this cellular population, in vivo and in vitro, is the most convincing evidence of the properties of cancer stem cells. To islolate and study this population, primary tumor masses are reduced into single cell suspensions, FACs sorted into different subpopulations using cell surface markers and subsequently injected in NOD-SCID recipient animals. These cells can also be grown as spheres *in vitro* under non-adherent conditions to enrich the CSC population. The CSC cells should be able to re-establish the phenotypes associated with the donor tumor and exhibit self-renewing capacity upon serial passaging. It is easier to work with leukemic stem cells as they have defined surface markers; however the surface markers have not been clearly defined in the solid tumors and makes it difficult to isolate this subpopulation with ease. Over the years accumulating data suggests a number of cell surface markers that have been characterized and have proven helpful in isolation of this cellular population. Surface antigens such as CD133, CD44, CD24 and ABC transporters have been used to isolate putative CSCs from tumors and grown *in vitro*. Interestingly growth of tumor cells *in vitro* as spheres/spheroids allows enrichment of this subpopulation. In breast cancers $CD44^{+}/CD24^{-/low}$ cells have been shown to successfully form tumors and elicit stem cell like phenotype [3]. This was the first evidence of isolation of putative cancer stem cells from solid tumor. Thereafter, CD133 was used to isolate this cellular population from brain tumors (glioblastoma multiforme and medulloblastoma) [2]. CD133 was also used to isolate the cells from colon carcinoma [4]. In head and neck carcinoma, $CD44^+$ cells were isolated as putative cancer stem cell which formed 0.1-42% of the tumors cells and successfully formed tumors when transplanted in NOD/SCID subcutaneously [10]. $CD133^+$ and $CD44^+/CD24^+/ESA^+$ cells with tumorigenic properties were isolated from pancreas, similarly, $CD133^+$ cells in lung carcinoma and $CD90^+$ cell in liver tumor were found to have potential cancer stem cell properties [11]. Interestingly one observes non-uniformity within the same cancer subtypes. Two distinct populations were found within BRCA1-deficient mouse mammary tumors. There was $CD44^+/CD24^-$ and $CD133^+$ populations which were independently tumorigenic in NOD/SCID mice but did not overlap between themselves [12]. Work by Joo and colleagues show that though $CD133^+$ cells from glioblastoma cells can initiate tumor, the $CD133^-$ population also possesses tumor-initiating properties [13] contrary to reports from other tumors suggesting that only $CD133^+$ cells are tumor-initiating. Similarly in colon cancer $CD133^-$ cells can also give rise to tumor in NOD/SCID mice [14]. Thus the use of cell surface markers for isolation of cancer stem cells has complexity to it and may cause impedence to identification of tumor-initiating population for therapy.

Are the Cancer Stem Cells, the Metastatic Cells?

Metastasis of tumors is the cause of lethality in cancer patients. However not all the cells in a tumor metastasize and neither do they all have the capability to metastasize. To metastasize, cells require a panorama of cellular changes such as self-sufficient growth signals, resistance to programmed death and anoikis, insensitivity to growth inhibitory signals, limitless self replicative potential and ability to initiate angiogenesis. In epithelial solid tumors the cells require to undergo transition to become mesenchymal and acquire phenotypes capable of aiding invasion [15]. A recent report suggests that there may be a direct link between acquisition of stem cell properties and EMT [16]. Mani and colleagues show that transformed human mammary epithelial cells that have undergone EMT formed tumors efficiently and also stem-like cells islolated from the mammary tumors expressed EMT markers. A similar report suggests that cells possessing both stemness and tumorigenicity can be derived from human mammary epithelial cells following Ras-MAPK activation and acquisition of these characteristics is driven by EMT induction [17]. $CD44^+$ cells from prostrate cancer, the CSC cellular population, were found to be more invasive and the genomic profile of these cells resembled that of $CD44^+/CD24^-$ prostrate CSC cells. These were more tumorigenic in NOD/SCID suggesting that metastasis may be mediated by the potential CSCs [18]. Another report which provides support to the concept of metastatic cancer stem cells is from pancreatic cancer. It shows that $CD133^+/CXCR4^+$ CSCs were found at the invasive front of pancreatic tumors and possessed strong migratory activity. Interestingly, only $CD133^+CXCR4^+$ cells metastasized to the liver *in vivo* and depletion of this population affected tumorigenic potential suggesting the existence of a CSC pool which possesses metastatic potential [19]. Similarly in osteocarcinoma, Berman et al. showed that Sca-1 positive population was highly proliferative, retained tumorigenic potential and formed metastatic tumors indicating a correlation between the stemness and metastasis [20]. Collectively these findings suggest an existence or generation of a sub-population of tumor cells which bear both metastatic and stem cell properties. If this hypothesis is true then it can contribute to a new generation of therapeutic drugs which can target this metastatic cancer stem cell population.

Pathways in Cancer Stem Cells

Since cancer stem cells possess the ability to self-renew it can be expected to find signaling pathways regulating the self-renewal to be operational in them. Signaling pathways, associated with carcinogenesis such as WNT and Notch, may also regulate stem cell self-renewal [21, 22]. Notch signaling is oncogenic and contributes to carcinoma progression in various carcinomas [23] similarly WNT signaling is also implicated in carcinoma progression [24] (figure 1).

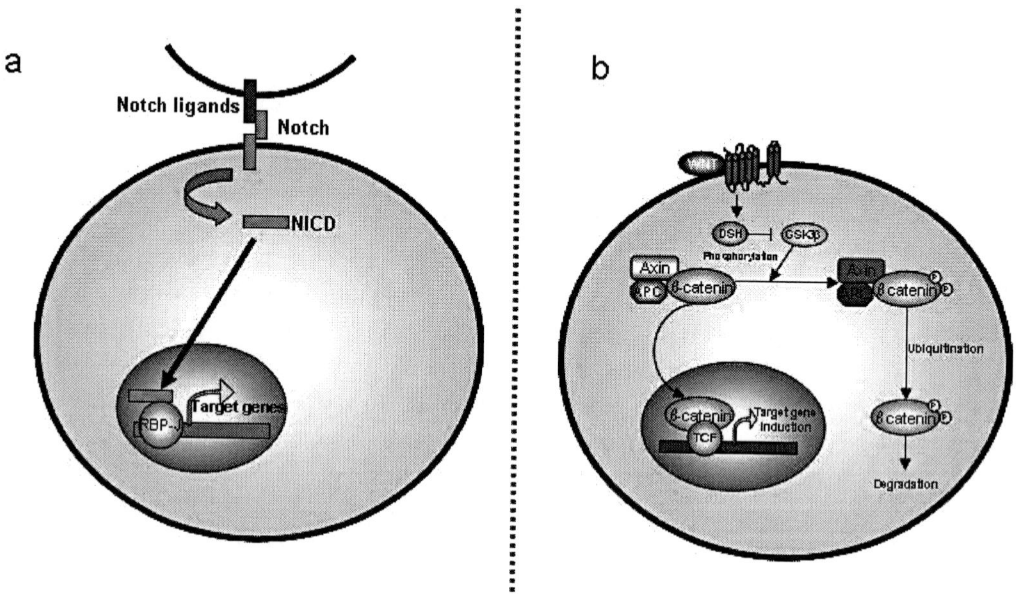

Figure 1. (a) simplified diagram of canonical notch and wnt signaling pathway. (a) Activation of Notch upon ligand receptor interaction results in formation of Notch intracellular domain (NICD), after sequential proteolytic steps. The NICD translocates to the nucleus, where it binds RBP-J resulting in expression of target genes including Hes1. (b) During Wnt signaling, binding of Wnt to frizzled results in inactivation of degradation complex, allowing accumulation of b-catenin which subsequently enters the nucleus. In the nucleus it binds with other proteins including Tcf to form a complex, which leads to transcriptional regulation of Wnt genes including c-Myc. Abbreviations: GSK3b-glycogen synthase kinase 3b; APC-adenomatous polyposis coli.

Notch receptor is a single-pass transmembrane receptor and is activated upon cleavage to form active intracellular domain. Ligand (Jagged and Delta) binding to the receptor triggers Notch activation resulting in cleaved intracellular domain. Notch signaling has been implicated in development and cell fate determination for decades [25]. Further Artavanis-Tsakonas and co-workers first established the possible involvement of Notch in human solid tumors. Aberrant Notch1 signaling was observed in cervical carcinomas with prominent expression of intracellular Notch1 domain [26]. Subsequently Daniel et al (1997) reported that greater Notch1 expression was observed in invasive cervical carcinomas as opposed to high-grade lesions [27]. Notch signaling is also aberrantly activated in other human malignancies [28, 29]. The co-operative transformation with papillomavirus oncogenes E6 and E7, induction of anoikis resistance, inhibition of p53 and upregulation of myc are important features attributed to Notch signaling associated with cervical cancer progression [30-36]. Aberrant Notch signaling also induces cyclin D1 and CDK2 activity [37]. Reports suggest that Notch signaling affects mammalian stem cells including hematopoietic stem cell [38]. Interestingly aberrant Notch signaling has also been implicated in cancer stem cells.

Notch expression has been observed in $CD44^{+}CD24^{-}$ and $CD133^{+}$ breast cancer cells which also express Sox1 and Oct4 [12]. Study with human glioma cell lines showed moderate to high expression levels of Notch receptors and ligands [5]. Overexpression of activated Notch1 in glioma cell lines resulted in increased neurosphere-like colonies which expressed Nestin and could undergo differentiation. This data suggests the role of Notch signaling in formation of cancer stem-like cells in human gliomas. In another report, Dontu and colleagues show that Notch activation using Dsl peptides resulted in increased secondary mammosphere formation [39]. The involvement of Notch1 in cancer stem cells can also be highlighted from the work of Farnie and Clarke who showed that $CD44^{+}CD24^{-}$ cells had Notch genes upregulated, and gamma-secretase inhibitor, DAPT, reduced DCIS mammosphere formation, indicating that Notch signaling is essential for stem cell self-renewal [40]. In another interesting observation by Fan et al. inhibition of Notch signaling reduced the $CD133^{+}$ cell fraction by 5-fold totally abolishing the side population, suggesting that the loss of tumor-forming capacity could be due to the depletion of stem-like cells [41].

Another signaling pathway that is involved in cell fate determination is the Wnt pathway. Wnt signaling is regulated by beta-catenin. When Wnt signaling is absent beta-catenin is rapidly degraded following its phosphorylation by GSK3beta in the presence of activated APC complex. Upon initiation of Wnt signaling the beta-catenin phosphorylation is inhibited and the latter accumulates in the nucleus. It binds with TCF/LEF family and result in transcriptional upregulation of genes [42]. Wnt signaling has been shown to play a role in hematopoietic self-renewal, and experimental evidence from transgenic mouse models has shown that activation of the Wnt signaling pathway in stem cells can lead to epithelial tumors [22]. Studies in gut morphogenesis suggest that Wnt signaling plays and important role in cell fate determination and morphogenesis [43]. Wnt signaling also contributes to tumorigenesis and stem cell renewal [44]. Results suggest that overexpression of Wnt in mouse mammary glands led to increased mammary tumor formation [45]. In a recent study activation of WNT signaling in CD133+ cells, containing Cre-dependent mutant allele of beta-catenin, resulted in expansion of CD133+ cells [46]. Taken together, these observations suggest that Notch pathway and WNT signaling play important roles in cancer stem-like cells and appear to be a legitimate target for cancer therapy.

Therapeutic Implications

According to the clonal evolution model, transformation results from random mutation and subsequent clonal selection. In this model, any cell may be the target of carcinogenesis while the stem cell model of carcinogenesis suggests that cancers originate in tissue stem cells or progenitor cells probably through dysregulation of self-renewal or signaling pathways.

This leads to expansion of this cell population that may undergo further genetic or epigenetic changes to become fully transformed. Both models of cancer progression are most likely to exist in a cancer. In recent past several new anti-cancer drugs have been introduced however the survival rates have not seen a drastic change. Radiation therapy or chemotherapy can completely destroy the primary tumor but there is usually a relapse of cancer along with metastasis. Even if the present therapies cause complete regression of tumors, they may not eliminate a population of cell which is chemotherapy or radiotherapy resistant that may survive longer to cause relapse. Reports suggest that the quiescent CSCs are more resistant to chemotherapy and radiation therapy. Bao et al showed that CD133 expressing brain CSCs were enriched upon radiation therapy. An expansion of $CD133^+$ cellular population both *in vivo* and *in vitro* suggested that the CSC population is resistant to ionizing radiation. These cells expectedly activated the DNA damage checkpoint response effectively as compared to $CD133^-$ cells, thus conferring resistant property [47]. Similarly pancreatic carcinoma $CD133^+$ subpopulation showed resistance to gemcitabine, a drug used for pancreatic cancer treatment [19]. In another study, Woodward and colleagues showed that the progenitors in the murine mammary epithelial cell cultures were enriched upon exposure to ionizing radiation. Interestingly they observed that the enrichment was enhanced by beta-catenin stabilization [48]. If one is to believe that the growth of solid tumor is driven by cancer stem cells, then CSCs have a very important implication in terms of future cancer treatment and therapies. Present cancer therapy treats the tumor as a bulk irrespective of the fact that they have diverse cell types. In contrast to cancer cells, cancer stem cells are slow-dividing, quiescent, have increased ability of DNA repair and are resistant to chemotherapy and radiation [49]. Ishikawa and colleagues show that leukemic stem cells, with self-renewal properties, home to bone marrow when xenotransplanted. These cells are protected from chemotherapy induced cell death. Similarly the $CD44^+CD24^{-/low}$ cells from breast carcinoma showed radiation resistant properties [50]. Phillips and colleagues showed that irradiating $CD24^{-/low}/CD44^+$ cancer-initiating cells isolated from MCF-7 and MDA-MB-231 resulted in relatively increased numbers of radioresistant population. These cells were more resistant than cells grown as monolayer cultures and had higher Notch1 activation and clonogenic survival properties. The potential enrichment of this subpoplation during radiation and chemotherapy suggests their implication in tumor progression and relapse and the need to target therapy towards this population.

The cancer stem cells not only have increased DNA repair but also express multidrug resistant genes which protects them against cytotoxic agents [51, 52]. The mechanism underlying drug resistance is not clearly defined but stem cells express various multi-drug resistant proteins such as multi-drug resistance protein1 (MDR1) which may contribute to drug resistance. Current therapeutic strategies use specific markers such as the mutated or overexpressed proteins in a tumor cell to develop anti-cancer drugs. However this approach is again yielding complete remission. Example includes, traztuzamab, a monoclonal antibody developed to target ErbB2 oncogene, which is overexpressed in only a subset of breast cancer, does not cause complete tumor remission. Thus it might be more rewarding to also target stem cell maintenance signaling pathways as therapeutic targets. However it needs to be selectively targeted without affecting the normal stem cell. Ito and colleagues showed that the generally quiescent leukemia-initiating cells can be targeted for therapy using a tumor suppressor called promyelocytic leukemia protein (PML) [53]. Chronic myeloid leukemia is a typical hematopoietic stem cell disease in which the leukemia-initiating-cells are not eradicated by current therapy resulting in relapse of disease. The present observation with PML provides hope for targeting quiescent leukemia-initiating cells to achieve complete cure. In another recent finding, targeting of CSCs showed very encouraging observation. L1CAM, neuronal cell adhesion molecule with higher expression in the $CD133^+$ cells as compared to $CD133^-$ glioma cells, was abolished using shRNA. L1CAM regulates the expression of p21(WAF1/CIP1) tumor suppressor and Olig2, thus its ablation resulted in disruption in neurosphere formation, induction of apoptosis in glioma cells and decreased tumor formation [47].

Interestingly Michael Clarke and colleagues have provided new data that reaffirms radioresistant property attributed to CSCs. They describe a mechanism that may address the question- how CSCs resist radiotherapy. They measured the intracellular concentrations of pro-oxidants and found that ROS levels were low in CSCs. The ROS related genes were expressed more highly in $CD44^+/CD24^{-/low}/Lin^-$ cells as compared to non-tumorigenic cells. They were also able to radiosensitize CSCs by inhibiting the enzymes involved in glutathione synthesis, a key antioxidant [54]. Taken together these studies suggest a possible role of CSCs in radiotherapy resistance. Drug therapy targeted for cancer treatment will thus need to meet the objective of possible elimination of this cellular population.

The studies by Phillips et al. and Bao et al. have important clinical implications as they clearly identify CSCs which are radiotherapy resistant and support the idea of possible relapse of tumor due to CSCs. The need of the hour is to develop radio/chemosensitizers that can lead to preferential sensitization of this subpopulation followed by complete elimination.

Conclusion

There is accumulating evidence for the existence of cancer stem cells in human carcinomas. Use of surface markers has led to isolation of a subpopulation in tumor which has both tumorigenic and self-renewal properties. However identification of this population is complex in solid-tumors due to heterogeneity (between tumors and within tumors) and lack of surface markers. Even within a given tumor there is poor overlap with subsequent identification of more than one population. It will be necessary to do gene expression profiling or proteomic analysis of various tumors and their subsets to establish specific cell surface antigens. A successful approach to isolation of CSC may also require a genetic profiling of the normal stem cells and a comparison between the normal and CSCs. Thus it is imperative that accurate identification of tumor-initiating population must be made in tumor specific manner before treatment is initiated. Though the frequency of CSCs varies between tumors and subtypes, nonetheless the existence of CSCs is irrefutable and their contribution to chemotherapy resistance and radiotherapy resistance is an interesting field to be exploited to ensure complete cure. In light of the accumulating data and current studies it is becoming clear that identification of CSCs and characterization of these for every tumor will help in designing personalized and tumor specific new therapies. The recent finding by Diehn et al. is an interesting beginning in this field as it suggests one of the possible mechanisms that may allow the CSCs to gain resistance. The gain of resistance, escape from radiation and chemotherapy and relapse seem to be properties of CSCs that needs to be addressed for complete cure of cancer. It is thus increasingly important to decipher the other mechanisms of resistance of CSCs to chemotherapy and radiotherapy. As the signaling pathway directed drugs and cytotoxic drugs have not been able to cause complete remission of cancer it will be necessary to introduce combinatorial regimen which includes both cytotoxic drugs and targeted therapies against CSCs for complete elimination of this population and prevention of relapse (figure 2).

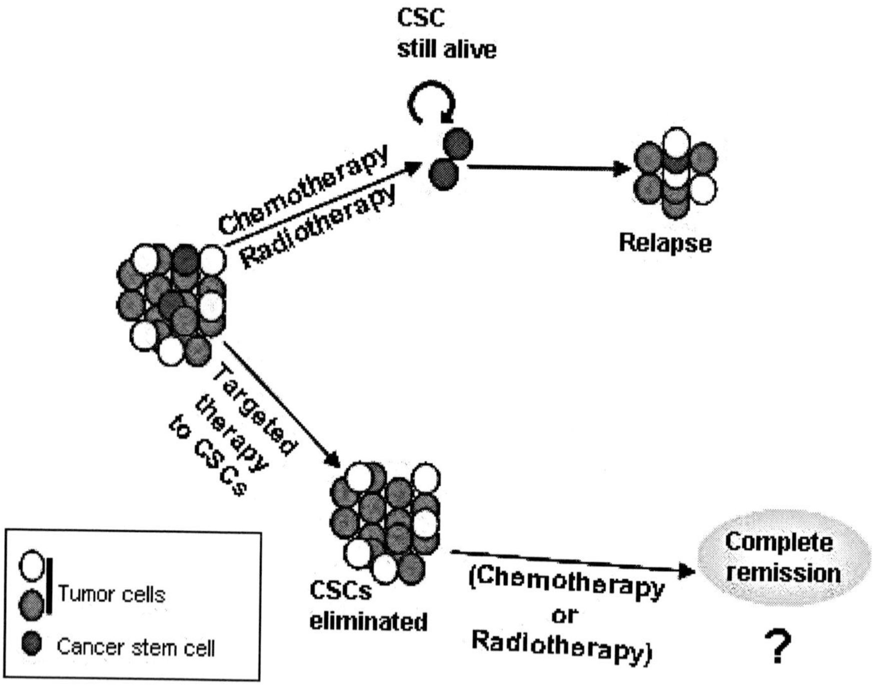

Figure 2. Current therapy leads to killing of tumor cells but complete remission does not happen. If the cancer stem cells are radioresistant and chemoresistant then they remain viable for prolonged period and re-establish tumors. If, however according to the recent therapeutic approach, the tumor was targeted for CSCs first then it may allow for killing of all the tumor cells including CSCs allowing for complete remission.

References

[1] Bonnet, D. and J.E. Dick, Human acute myeloid leukemia is organized as a hierarchy that originates from a primitive hematopoietic cell. *Nat .Med*, 1997. 3(7): p. 730-7.

[2] Singh, S.K., et al., Cancer stem cells in nervous system tumors. *Oncogene,* 2004. 23(43): p. 7267-73.

[3] Al-Hajj, M., et al., Prospective identification of tumorigenic breast cancer cells. *Proc. Natl. Acad. Sci. USA,* 2003. 100(7): p. 3983-8.

[4] O'Brien, C.A., et al., A human colon cancer cell capable of initiating tumour growth in immunodeficient mice. *Nature*, 2007. 445(7123): p. 106-10.

[5] Zhang, S., et al., Identification and characterization of ovarian cancer-initiating cells from primary human tumors. *Cancer Res,* 2008. 68(11): p. 4311-20.

[6] Li, C., et al., Identification of pancreatic cancer stem cells. *Cancer Res,* 2007. 67(3): p. 1030-7.

[7] Lang, S.H., F.M. Frame, and A.T. Collins, Prostate cancer stem cells. *J. Pathol*, 2009. 217(2): p. 299-306.

[8] Maitland, N.J. and A.T. Collins, Prostate cancer stem cells: a new target for therapy. *J. Clin. Oncol,* 2008. 26(17): p. 2862-70.

[9] Krivtsov, A.V., et al., Transformation from committed progenitor to leukaemia stem cell initiated by MLL-AF9. *Nature,* 2006. 442(7104): p. 818-22.

[10] Prince, M.E., et al., Identification of a subpopulation of cells with cancer stem cell properties in head and neck squamous cell carcinoma. *Proc. Natl. Acad. Sci. USA*, 2007. 104(3): p. 973-8.

[11] Eramo, A., et al., Identification and expansion of the tumorigenic lung cancer stem cell population. *Cell Death Differ,* 2008. 15(3): p. 504-14.

[12] Wright, M.H., et al., Brca1 breast tumors contain distinct CD44+/CD24- and CD133+ cells with cancer stem cell characteristics. *Breast Cancer Res*, 2008. 10(1): p. R10.

[13] Joo, K.M., et al., Clinical and biological implications of CD133-positive and CD133-negative cells in glioblastomas. *Lab Invest*, 2008. 88(8): p. 808-15.

[14] Shmelkov, S.V., et al., CD133 expression is not restricted to stem cells, and both CD133+ and CD133- metastatic colon cancer cells initiate tumors. *J. Clin. Invest*, 2008. 118(6): p. 2111-20.

[15] Thiery, J.P., Epithelial-mesenchymal transitions in tumour progression. *Nat. Rev. Cancer*, 2002. 2(6): p. 442-54.

[16] Mani, S.A., et al., The epithelial-mesenchymal transition generates cells with properties of stem cells. *Cell,* 2008. 133(4): p. 704-15.

[17] Morel, A.P., et al., Generation of breast cancer stem cells through epithelial-mesenchymal transition. *PLoS ONE*, 2008. 3(8): p. e2888.

[18] Klarmann, G.J., et al., Invasive prostate cancer cells are tumor initiating cells that have a stem cell-like genomic signature. *Clin. Exp. Metastasis*, 2009.

[19] Hermann, P.C., et al., Distinct populations of cancer stem cells determine tumor growth and metastatic activity in human pancreatic cancer. *Cell Stem Cell*, 2007. 1(3): p. 313-23.

[20] Berman, S.D., et al., Metastatic osteosarcoma induced by inactivation of Rb and p53 in the osteoblast lineage. *Proc. Natl. Acad. Sci. USA*, 2008. 105(33): p. 11851-6.

[21] Stier, S., et al., Notch1 activation increases hematopoietic stem cell self-renewal in vivo and favors lymphoid over myeloid lineage outcome. *Blood,* 2002. 99(7): p. 2369-78.

[22] Reya, T., et al., A role for Wnt signalling in self-renewal of haematopoietic stem cells. *Nature*, 2003. 423(6938): p. 409-14.

[23] Maliekal, T.T., et al., The role of Notch signaling in human cervical cancer: implications for solid tumors. *Oncogene*, 2008. 27(38): p. 5110-4.

[24] Katoh, M., WNT/PCP signaling pathway and human cancer (review). *Oncol. Rep.*, 2005. 14(6): p. 1583-8.

[25] Greenwald, I., LIN-12/Notch signaling: lessons from worms and flies. *Genes Dev*, 1998. 12(12): p. 1751-62.

[26] Zagouras, P., et al., Alterations in Notch signaling in neoplastic lesions of the human cervix. *Proc. Natl. Acad. Sci. USA,* 1995. 92(14): p. 6414-8.

[27] Daniel, B., et al., The link between integration and expression of human papillomavirus type 16 genomes and cellular changes in the evolution of cervical intraepithelial neoplastic lesions. *J. Gen. Virol*, 1997. 78 (Pt 5): p. 1095-101.

[28] Farnie, G., et al., Novel cell culture technique for primary ductal carcinoma in situ: role of Notch and epidermal growth factor receptor signaling pathways. *J. Natl. Cancer Inst*, 2007. 99(8): p. 616-27.

[29] Miyamoto, Y., et al., Notch mediates TGF alpha-induced changes in epithelial differentiation during pancreatic tumorigenesis. *Cancer Cell*, 2003. 3(6): p. 565-76.

[30] Rangarajan, A., et al., Activated Notch1 signaling cooperates with papillomavirus oncogenes in transformation and generates resistance to apoptosis on matrix withdrawal through PKB/Akt. *Virology*, 2001. 286(1): p. 23-30.

[31] Weng, A.P., et al., c-Myc is an important direct target of Notch1 in T-cell acute lymphoblastic leukemia/lymphoma. *Genes Dev*, 2006. 20(15): p. 2096-109.

[32] Klinakis, A., et al., Myc is a Notch1 transcriptional target and a requisite for Notch1-induced mammary tumorigenesis in mice. *Proc. Natl. Acad. Sci. USA*, 2006. 103(24): p. 9262-7.

[33] Kim, S.B., et al., Activated Notch1 interacts with p53 to inhibit its phosphorylation and transactivation. *Cell Death Differ,* 2006.

[34] Subramanyam, D. and S. Krishna, c-Myc substitutes for Notch1-CBF1 functions in cooperative transformation with papillomavirus oncogenes. *Virology,* 2006. 347(1): p. 191-8.

[35] Nair, P., K. Somasundaram, and S. Krishna, Activated Notch1 inhibits p53-induced apoptosis and sustains transformation by human papillomavirus type 16 E6 and E7 oncogenes through a PI3K-PKB/Akt-dependent pathway. *J. Virol*, 2003. 77(12): p. 7106-12.

[36] Lathion, S., et al., Notch1 can contribute to viral-induced transformation of primary human keratinocytes. *Cancer Res,* 2003. 63(24): p. 8687-94.

[37] Ronchini, C. and A.J. Capobianco, Induction of cyclin D1 transcription and CDK2 activity by Notch(ic): implication for cell cycle disruption in transformation by Notch(ic). *Mol. Cell Biol.*, 2001. 21(17): p. 5925-34.

[38] Radtke, F., et al., The role of Notch signaling during hematopoietic lineage commitment. *Immunol. Rev.*, 2002. 187: p. 65-74.

[39] Dontu, G., et al., Role of Notch signaling in cell-fate determination of human mammary stem/progenitor cells. *Breast Cancer Res.*, 2004. 6(6): p. R605-15.

[40] Farnie, G. and R.B. Clarke, Mammary stem cells and breast cancer--role of Notch signalling. *Stem Cell Rev*, 2007. 3(2): p. 169-75.

[41] Fan, X., et al., Notch pathway inhibition depletes stem-like cells and blocks engraftment in embryonal brain tumors. *Cancer Res.*, 2006. 66(15): p. 7445-52.

[42] Wodarz, A. and R. Nusse, Mechanisms of Wnt signaling in development. *Annu. Rev. Cell Dev. Biol.*, 1998. 14: p. 59-88.

[43] Theodosiou, N.A. and C.J. Tabin, Wnt signaling during development of the gastrointestinal tract. *Dev. Biol*, 2003. 259(2): p. 258-71.

[44] Li, Y., et al., Evidence that transgenes encoding components of the Wnt signaling pathway preferentially induce mammary cancers from progenitor cells. *Proc. Natl. Acad. Sci. USA*, 2003. 100(26): p. 15853-8.

[45] Schroeder, J.A., et al., ErbB-beta-catenin complexes are associated with human infiltrating ductal breast and murine mammary tumor virus (MMTV)-Wnt-1 and MMTV-c-Neu transgenic carcinomas. *J. Biol. Chem*, 2002. 277(25): p. 22692-8.

[46] Zhu, L., et al., Prominin 1 marks intestinal stem cells that are susceptible to neoplastic transformation. *Nature,* 2009. 457(7229): p. 603-7.

[47] Bao, S., et al., Glioma stem cells promote radioresistance by preferential activation of the DNA damage response. *Nature,* 2006. 444(7120): p. 756-60.

[48] Woodward, W.A., et al., WNT/beta-catenin mediates radiation resistance of mouse mammary progenitor cells. *Proc. Natl. Acad. Sci. USA*, 2007. 104(2): p. 618-23.

[49] Ishikawa, F., et al., Chemotherapy-resistant human AML stem cells home to and engraft within the bone-marrow endosteal region. *Nat. Biotechnol*, 2007. 25(11): p. 1315-21.

[50] Phillips, T.M., W.H. McBride, and F. Pajonk, The response of CD24(-/low)/CD44+ breast cancer-initiating cells to radiation. *J. Natl. Cancer Inst*, 2006. 98(24): p. 1777-85.

[51] Lu, C. and A. Shervington, Chemoresistance in gliomas. *Mol. Cell Biochem.*, 2008. 312(1-2): p. 71-80.

[52] Zhou, S., et al., The ABC transporter Bcrp1/ABCG2 is expressed in a wide variety of stem cells and is a molecular determinant of the side-population phenotype. *Nat. Med*, 2001. 7(9): p. 1028-34.

[53] Ito, K., et al., PML targeting eradicates quiescent leukaemia-initiating cells. *Nature*, 2008. 453(7198): p. 1072-8.

[54] Diehn, M., et al., Association of reactive oxygen species levels and radioresistance in cancer stem cells. *Nature,* 2009.

In: Stem Cell Therapy and Uses in Medical Treatment
Editor: Prasad S. Koka, pp. 117-141
ISBN: 978-1-61324-008-3

Chapter 8

Rescue of Multi-lineage Hematopoiesis during HIV-1 Infection by Human c-mpl Gene Transfer and Reconstitution of CD34+ Progenitor Cells *In Vivo*

Menghua Zhang[1], Tuang Yeow Poh[1], Fawzia Louache[2,3,4,5], I. Birgitta Sundell[1], Jinyun Yuan[1], Stella Evans[1] and Prasad S. Koka*[1]

[1]Laboratory of Stem Cell Biology, Torrey Pines Institute for Molecular Studies, 3550 General Atomics Court, San Diego, California 92121, USA;

[2] Institut National de la Santé et de la Recherche Médicale U790, Villejuif;

[3] Institut Gustave Roussy, IFR54, Villejuif;

[4] Université Paris VII, Paris; [5] Université Paris XI, Villejuif; France

Abstract

Cytopenias arising from hematopoietic abnormalities are a severe common complication contributing to early mortality in HIV/AIDS patients. The proto-oncogene *c-mpl,* identified as the thrombopoietin receptor is involved in multilineage differentiation of CD34+ hematopoietic progenitor cells. We have introduced the *c-mpl* gene into CD34+ cells via transduction of the lentivirus p156RRLsinPPTmPGK-CMPL-PRE. The lentiviral construct expresses c-mpl on approximately 90% of purified CD34+ cells. These transduced cells have then been reconstituted into human fetal thymus/liver implants in severe combined immunodeficient mice (SCID-hu Thy/Liv). The c-mpl expression on transduced CD34+ cells is not susceptible to downregulation due to the effects of HIV-1 infection. Reconstituted CD34+ cells transduced with control lentivirus,

* Corresponding Author: Prasad S. Koka, PhD Associate Member, Laboratory of Stem Cell Biologyl Torrey Pines Institute for Molecular Studies, 3550 General Atomics Court, San Diego, CA 92121. Tel (858) 597 3886. Fax (858) 597 3804. Email pkoka@tpims.org

p156RRLsinPPTmPGK-EGFP-PRE, express EGFP at >90%. Reconstituted c-mpl expressing SCID-hu implants show almost maximum rescue (~90%) of myelopoiesis, erythropoiesis and megakaryopoiesis, during HIV-1 infection *in vivo*, at 6 weeks post-infection. We also show that the differentiated multi-lineage progeny colonies and thymocytes in mice reconstituted with the c-mpl transduced CD34+ cells, carry the HLA Class I loci phenotypes of these donor cells, in the implants of the recipient SCID-hu animals. We propose a gene therapeutic strategy, with *c-mpl* as the major genetic component, to address the morbidity and mortality resulting from cytopenias in HIV infected patients.

Keywords: HIV, SCID-hu, Hematopoiesis, Resurgence.

Introduction

HIV infected patients often suffer from multiple hematopoietic abnormalities which include anemia, thrombocytopenia, lymphocytopenia, monocytopenia, neutropenia, and myelodysplastic / hyperplastic alterations of the bone marrow microenvironment [1, 2]. Cytopenias are also induced by continued AZT treatment or HAART of HIV infected patients [3, 4], with thrombocytopenia more persistent than the other cytopenias [1]. Thrombocytopenia can present a greater risk for HIV infected individuals receiving HAART and who also require cardiovascular surgery [5]. The factors which could play a role in HIV mediated hematopoietic inhibition include direct intracellular effects of virus infection, interactions with viral proteins at the cell surface, and perturbation of cytokine network due to abnormal expression of cellular genes. The products of these genes could include growth factor receptors, receptor tyrosine kinases and factors involved in embryonic development, or immune mediated effects.

It has been observed that hematopoietic progenitor cell colony growth and differentiation is inhibited in long-term bone marrow cultures of HIV positive patients [6-9]. In general, investigators have failed to detect HIV infection in hematopoietic progenitor cells isolated from infected individuals, suggesting that HIV might have an indirect effect on hematopoiesis [10]. Although infection of CD34+ progenitor cells in vitro has been reported by some investigators [11, 12], the majority of studies found that bone marrow and peripheral blood derived CD34+ progenitor cells are not susceptible to HIV-1 infection in vitro [2, 13, 14]. Our own studies confirm the resistance of CD34+ cells to HIV-1 infection [15]. It has further been reported that primitive hematopoietic cells resist HIV-1 infection via $p21^{Waf1/Cip1/Sdi}$ [16]. HIV-1 inhibits multilineage hematopoiesis in vivo without direct infection of the CD34+ progenitor cells, and presumably via indirect effects of the infected microenvironment [15, 17]. These results suggest that HIV possibly alters the stromal / progenitor cell micro-environment that supports hematopoiesis. Our earlier studies revealed that the resurgence of colony forming units (CFU) following HIV-1 induced hematopoietic inhibition due to treatment with combination antiretroviral drugs is only transient [18]. The findings of other investigators showed that these drugs induce cytopenias in HIV infected individuals [3, 4].

The proto-oncogene, *c-mpl*, identified as the thrombopoietin (Tpo) receptor, is known to promote multi-lineage stem cell differentiation of the CD34+ progenitor cells [19-23]. Therefore we propose that *c-mpl* is an important target gene for control and enhancement of multi-lineage stem cell differentiation to reduce or prevent cytopenias arising from hematopoietic inhibition induced during HIV infection. To test this hypothesis, we used the severe combined immunodeficient mouse co-transplanted with human fetal thymus and liver tissues (SCID-hu Thy/Liv), wherein a conjoint hematopoietic organ develops. This is a very useful and well established small chimeric animal model system, which facilitates the investigation of the mechanisms of, and therapies for HIV induced hematopoietic inhibition [15, 18, 24]. This model system not only mimics HIV infection but also recapitulates functional human hematopoiesis in vivo [25]. The effects of HIV that are seen in this model are the direct result of virus mediated phenomena. Using the SCID-hu model, we have found that HIV-1 mediates hematopoietic inhibition in vivo, as assessed by multi-lineage CFU of the CD34+ progenitor cells derived from the Thy/Liv implants [18]. We and others have reported that the colony forming activity/units of the CD34+ cells derived from HIV-1 infected patients is reduced or inhibited, suggesting that there are indirect effects of HIV-1 on CD34+ cells that persist ex vivo [7, 8, 26, 27, 25]. This is accompanied by a decrease in c-mpl expression of the CD34+ cells [28]. Herein we show that stable restoration of c-mpl expression by placing the c-mpl gene under the control of a housekeeping gene promoter produces a substantial and sustained rescue of hematopoiesis, during HIV-1 infection.

Materials and Methods

Cell culture. 293T cells were grown in Dulbecco`s modified Eagle`s medium (DMEM) containing 10%(v/v) fetal bovine serum (FBS), penicillin (100U/ml), streptomycin (100 □g/ml) and 2mM L-glutamine. 293T cells are used for preparation of lentivirus.

Primary human CD34+ cell isolation from fetal liver and their culture. Primary human CD34+ hematopoietic progenitor cells were isolated from human fetal liver by Ficoll-Hypaque density gradient centrifugation followed by passage through Miltenyi Biotec AutoMacs CD34+ cell separation columns. Cells were used immediately after isolation or kept frozen at -80^0C and liquid N_2 for use at a later time.

Separation of CD34+CD38- cells into c-mpl+ and c-mpl- subsets. Purified CD34+ cells from the Thy/Liv implants were separated by AutoMacs into c-mpl+ and c-mpl- subsets. These subsets were subjected to two color FACS analyses, using anti-c-mpl-PE (BD Pharmingen, clone BAH-1) and anti-CD34-FITC monoclonal antibodies to estimate their purity.

HIV-1 viral stocks preparation. The CEM cell line was maintained in RPMI 1640 medium with 10% FBS (GIBCO, Invitrogen, U.S.A.). The cells were grown at 37°C in humidified incubator with 5% CO_2. Virus stocks of HIV-1 NL4-3 were produced by infecting CEM cells. Briefly, $10x10^6$ CEM cells were infected with 300-500ng/ml (p24 titer) of HIV-1 NL4-3 strain with 10μg polybrene in final 1 ml volume in 6-well plates at 37°C in 5% CO_2. The plate was shaken every half hour for 2-4 hours. After washing twice, cells were maintained in RPMI 1640 medium with 10% FBS. Viruses were collected at the peak of virus production (day 6 to 7) after centrifugation of the culture supernatants (800 x g for 10min), followed by filtration through 0.45-0.1μm pore size filters. Virus production was assessed by measuring p24 antigen concentrations using p24 ELISA (Perkin Elmer Life Sciences U.S.A.). Aliquots of viral stock were stored in -70°C.

Construction of chimeric SCID-hu (Thy/Liv) animals. SCID mice received simultaneous transplants of 1-3 mm pieces of human fetal thymus and liver of 18-24 weeks gestation (Advanced Bioscience Resources, Alameda, CA) under the renal capsule and the resulting conjoint organ was allowed to grow for 3-5 months to generate a SCID-hu animal [18, 25, 28].

Lentivirus preparation. Lentivirus containing supernatants were prepared by calcium phosphate-mediated cotransfection of 293T cells as previously described (using calcium phosphate transfection kit from Invitrogen Life Technologies, Carlsbad, CA) [29]. 293T cells were plated on poly-L-lysine-coated 10-cm plates at 5.5-6 x 10^6 cells per plate in DMEM with 10% FBS (D10) and allowed to adhere for 6-8 hrs before transfection. A mixture of three plasmid DNAs consisting of 10 μg transfer target [either c-mpl or EGFP, 10 μg of pCMVΔR8.2 for packaging, and 2 μg of pMD.G for pseudotyping with VSV-G envelope, were used for transfection of the 293T cells [30]. 8-12 hrs after application of the DNA precipitate, the cells were rinsed three times with PBS, and then subjected to induction in fresh D10 medium. Lentivirus supernatants were collected after 36-48 hrs incubation and then filtered through a 0.2 micron syringe filter and by ultracentrifugation at 50,000 x g for 2.5 hrs as previously described [31]. The p24 viral titer in lentivirus supernatant was determined by diagnostically certified p24 immunoassay (Perkin Elmer) according to the manufacturer's instructions. All p24 assays were performed in duplicate.

Cloning of human c-mpl gene into the self-inactivating lentiviral vector, p156RRLsinPPTmPGK-EGFP-PRE. The lentiviral plasmid, p156RRLsinPPTmPGK-EGFP-PRE, was digested with the restriction enzymes, NotI and XbaI to excise the EGFP gene, which was then replaced by the PCR amplified 1.9 kbp cDNA fragment of the *c-mpl* gene. The c-mpl cDNA clone wherein this gene was cloned into the XhoI site of pBluescript KS +/- vector, was provided by Dr. Francoise Wendling, Institut Gustave Roussy, France [32].

The human *c-mpl* gene cDNA was amplified from pBlueScript plasmid containing the *c-mpl* gene by using Invitrogen Platinum® PCR SuperMix High Fidelity by step-down PCR. The primers used were the sense primer (CMPL Forward 1) 5'-ATGTATC-CATATGATGCCCTCCTGGGCCCTCTTCATGGT-3' and the antisense primer (NotI CMPL Reverse) 5'- GCGGCCGCTTCAAGGCTGCTGCCAATAGCTTAGTGGTA-3'. Nested PCR was then carried out using 5 μl of the PCR products using the sense primer (CMPL Forward 2) 5'-GGATCCACCGGTCGCCACCATGTATCCATATGATGCCCTC-3' and the antisense primer (NotI CMPL Reverse) 5'- GCGGCCGCTT CAAGGC-TGCTGCCAATAGCTTAGTGGTA-3'. The PCR product was then TA cloned (Invitrogen Topo.TA cloning kit). The c-mpl cDNA was then excised from the TOPO vector with XbaI and NotI and then ligated into the same sites of a p156RRLsinPPTmPGK-EGFP-PRE vector containing an EGFP cDNA at those restriction sites, to generate a recombinant CMPL. Thermal cycle conditions are as follows: Initial denaturation at 94°C for 2 min, followed by 10 cycles of 94°C for 30 s, 68°C for 30 s (with decrement of 1°C per cycle) and 68°C for 1 ½ min and followed by 25 cycles of 94°C for 30 s, 58°C for 30 s and 68°C for 1 ½ min. *Restriction digestion:* The reaction mixture comprised approximately 5 μg of DNA, up to 10 U of restriction enzyme (ensuring final glycerol concentration was no more than 15% of total reaction volume), 2 μl of appropriate 10X reaction buffer (1X buffer) and sterile water up to a final volume of 20 μl. Digestion was carried out according to the manufacturer's instructions. The enzyme was then removed by using Qiagen PCR purification kit. *De-phosphorylation of vector:* The vector was digested with NotI and XbaI and purified as described above. The vector DNA was then de-phosphorylated with shrimp alkaline phosphatase (Promega). *Ligation of DNA into plasmid vector:* Excised fragments were ligated into the expression vector. The ligation reaction mix contained 20 U of T4 DNA ligase, 2 µl of 5X ligation buffer, and an appropriate volume of vector:insert ratio. The ligation reaction was then incubated overnight at 16°C.

C-mpl siRNA lentivirus construction. Lentiviral plasmids were obtained from addgene (www.addgene.com). They include pMD2.G, psPAX2, pLVTHM. Cmpl shRNA encoding primers up-stream, 5'-CGCGTCCCCTGACAGCATTATTCACATCTTCAAGAG AGATGT GAATAATGCTGTCATTTTTGGAAAT-3', down stream, 5'-CGATTTCCAAAAATGA CAGCATTATTCACATCTCTCTTGAAGATGTGAATAATGCTGTCAGGGGA -3' were designed targeting cmpl mRNA sequence TGACAGCATTATTCACATC. Double strand were generated by mixing equimolar amounts (100 µM) of two primers in annealing buffer (T4 ligase buffer) for 3 minute at 94°C, and slowly cooled to room temperature. Then it was directly inserted in the site of MluI and ClaI of the lentivector, pLVTHM, to generate CmplipLVTHM and then the plasmid was transformed into DH5α. Positive clones were screened by PCR for the correct insertion of hairpins and the sequence was verified.

C-mplipLVTHM plasmid was obtained using plasmid purification Maxi kit (Qiagen) according to manufacturer's instructions. Lentivirus was produced in human embryonic kidney 293T17 cells. 293T17 cells were seeded at 2.6×10^6 cells/10-cm dish, cultured for 24 h, and then transfected with 10 µg pLVTHM, 10 µg psPAX2, 2 µg pMDG.2 using Effectene transfection reagent (Invitrogen). Viruses were collected from cell culture media at 48 and 72 h after transfection and concentrated using SW-28 swinging bucket rotor at 25,000 rpm for 2 h. HIV-1 p24 antigen concentrations in the virus stocks were measured by an in-house p24 antigen enzyme-linked immunosorbent assay to evaluate the amount of input virus. To assess the knockdown of c-mpl gene, CD34+ hematopoietic progenitor cells were purified from human fetal liver using monoclonal antibody-conjugated immunomagnetic beads (Miltenyi Biotech, Auburn, CA, USA). The purity of CD34+ cells obtained was routinely >95%. Cells were cultured for one week in Iscove's medium containing 20% FBS and 10 ng/ml of each of the Stem Span cocktail cytokines Flt-3, IL-3, IL-6, and SCF. Culturing in Stem Span medium retained the immature CD34+CD38- phenotype. For vector transduction, CD34+ cells were incubated with the respective vectors for 2 hrs in the presence of 4µg/ml Polybrene. Two rounds of transductions were performed on 2 consecutive days. Transduced cells were examined by fluorescence microscope for EGFP expression 48-72 h posttransduction. The efficiency of c-mpl-specific RNAi was assayed by analyzing the expression of c-mpl-specific mRNA and c-mpl protein expression by FACS analysis. The c-mpl knocked down CD34+ cells were used for CFU both in vitro and in vivo.

Transduction of CD34+ cells with lentivirus expressing c-mpl and EGFP. Frozen CD34+ cells isolated from human fetal liver were thawed and plated at 1×10^5 cells per well on 24-well plates coated with fibronectin fragment CH-296 (TakaRa Bio, Otsu Shiga, Japan). The cells were pre-stimulated for 2-5 days in Stem Span H3000 serum-free medium with cytokine cocktail that contains Flt-3, SCF, IL-3, and IL-6 (all purchased from Stem Cell Technologies, Vancouver, BC, Canada). These pre-stimulated cells cultured in Stem Span retained the immature CD34+CD38- phenotype. Human CD34+ cells were transduced after pre-stimulation by adding lentivirus supernatants in the presence of Polybrene (4µg/ml). Twenty four hours after transduction, the medium was carefully removed and replaced by Iscove's modified Dulbecco's medium (IMDM), containing 20% FBS, with Stem Span cocktail cytokines. Cells were maintained in culture for 1 week after application of the lentivirus supernatant, at which time the cells were collected, washed with PBS and analyzed for c-mpl or EGFP expression by flow cytometry.

Construction and sequential biopsies of SCID-hu animals. SCID mice received simultaneous transplants of 1-mm^3 pieces of human fetal thymus and liver tissues under the renal capsule. The resulting conjoint organ of the SCID-hu animal was allowed to grow for 3 to 5 months, as described previously [28]. As necessary for analyses, sequential biopsies of the implants were performed at periodic intervals following mock, virus, or exogenous CD34+ cell injection and reconstitution.

Reconstitution of the SCID-hu implants. The above described construction of the SCID-hu animals consist of implants with the "endogenous" CD34+ cells. Injection of "exogenous" CD34+ cells into irradiated animals constitutes reconstitution. As relevant to the experiment, HIV-1 infection was carried out post-reconstitution.

HIV-1 or cloned lentivirus infection of SCID-hu animals. Thymocytes from the SCID-hu implants were infected through intra-implant injection with HIV1 NL4-3 (100 IU in 50-100ul). Control mock animals were injected with the same volume of mock infected cell culture medium. Lentivirus-transduced CD34+ cells were injected into the implants (1x10^4 cells / implant) of irradiated animals using EGFP-lentivirus as control for CMPL-lentivirus. A day later, exogenous untransduced or transduced CD34+ cell engrafted implants were infected with HIV-1.

Viral loads of the thymocytes of the Thy/Liv implants. HIV-1infectivity of the thymocytes of the Thy/Liv implants was determined by Quantitative (qt) PCR of the proviral DNA. qtPCR was performed using the kit Universal PCR Master Mix (Applied Biosystems) on an Applied Biosystems 7300 Real Time PCR machine. The following PCR primers were used: SR1: 5'-CCAGTAGTGTGTGCCCGTCTGT-3', and AA55: 5'-CTGCTAGAGATTTT CCACACTGAC-3', or 661: 5'-CCTGCGTCGAGAGAGCTCCTCTGG-3'. The probe 6FAM5' TGTGACTCTGGTAACTAGAGATCCCTCAGACCC-3'TAMRA was used in final 25μl reaction with cellular DNA. Primers were added at a final concentration of 900nM and the probe at a final concentration of 200nM. The reaction was incubated at 50°C 2 min., 95°C 10 min., then 45 cycles at 94°C 15 sec., 70°C 1 min., 72°C 1 min. β-globin was used as internal control. Its forward primer is: BGF1, 5'-CAACCTCAAACAGACACCATGG-3' and reverse primer BGR1, 5'-TCCACGTTCACCTTGCCC-3'. Threshold cycle (Ct) values of the target genes were normalized to the internal control genes. Differential expression in target samples relative to normal samples was calculated according to the 2-ΔΔCt method and manufacturer's directions.

Isolation of CD34+ CD38- cells from reconstituted SCID-hu Thy/Liv implants. We isolated the CD34+ cells from the mock- and HIV-1-infected Thy/Liv implants by labeling these cells with anti-CD34 monoclonal antibody (clone QBEND/10) conjugated to super paramagnetic MicroBeads (Miltenyi Biotec, Auburn, Calif.) and subjected to separation by AutoMacs (Miltenyi Biotec) using the "possel d2" software setting to maximize recovery and purity of the CD34+ cells. The separated CD34+CD38- cells were concentrated by centrifugation and relabeled with anti-CD34-allophycocyanin (APC) antibody (clone AC136, which recognizes a class III epitope of CD34 antigen; Miltenyi Biotec) for fluorescence-activated cell sorting (FACS) analysis for positive selection and to estimate purity. Cell surface expression of the CD38 antigen or the lack of it on the CD34+ cells is detected by dual or multi-color FACS analysis using the additional anti-CD38-FITC monoclonal antibody (clone IB6) purchased from Miltenyi Biotec. The purity of the CD34+ cells was estimated to be >95% by FACS analyses.

Hematopoietic colony forming unit (CFU) assays. As described previously 18, 28], myeloid and erythroid CFU of the purified CD34+ cells derived from Thy/Liv implants was determined by plating the cells in complete methylcellulose in the presence of hSCF, hGM-CSF, hIL-3, hEpo, or in megacult-C semi-solid media. Methylcellulose and megacult-C are purchased from Stem Cell Technologies, Vancouver, Canada. Megacult-C was used as recommended by the manufacturer. These assays were performed in duplicate, and the colonies were counted in the petri-dishes with grids by viewing them under the microscope.

Flow cytometry. FACS analyses were performed with the appropriately labeled monoclonal antibodies as described in the text or figure legends. Briefly, live cells were gated as determined by forward versus side scatter and analyzed using the CellQuest program (Becton Dickinson).

Transcripts of c-mpl. RNA was isolated from the CD34+ cells derived from the implants and converted to cDNA using the high fidelity polymerase. PCR was performed using the forward primer: 5'-GCAAGATGGACCAAAGCAGA-3', and the reverse primer: 5'-GCACTAGATGCAGAGCGGTC-3', with an expected c-mpl transcript of 829 bp. The reaction conditions were denaturation 94^0C 5 min, 32 cycles of 94^0C 1 min, 60^0C 1 min, and 72^0C 2 min denaturation, elongation and annealing, respectively, followed by 72^0C 7 min and cooling, 4^0C.

Statistical analyses. To compare groups we have used the Wilcoxon Rank Sum Test [24, 28], which is a nonparametric test that is powerful in small sample sizes. A Bonferroni-type correction was made to account for multiple comparisons. As replicated data can deflate the standard errors, we have averaged the replicates for each mouse so that the data retained their independence. *Power analysis.* It is estimated that after adjusting for multiple comparisons, the numbers of mice used have 80% power for an adjusted alpha level of 0.05 with a two-tailed test. We have used 4-6 animals in each experiment as required by these statistical analyses. The statistics with the p values as relevant are provided in the Table or Figure legends.

Results

Transfer of c-mpl gene into CD34+ cells via a lentiviral vector. The human c-mpl gene was placed under the control of the housekeeping murine phosphoglycerate kinase (mPGK) gene, promoter contained in a lentiviral vector, p156RRLsinPPTmPGK-EGFP-PRE, by substitution of the EGFP gene. This control lentiviral vector expressing EGFP and the p156RRLsinPPTmPGK-CMPL-PRE expressing c-mpl, were used for transduction of the human fetal CD34+ cells. The c-mpl- CD34+ cells, transduced with the lentivirus containing the c-mpl or control EGFP genes, were engrafted into the irradiated SCID-hu Thy/Liv implants.

Reconstitution of SCID-hu Thy/Liv implants by exogenous CD34+ cells: confirmation by HLA typing. The implants of these irradiated animals were reconstituted using untransduced or lentiviral transduced CD34+ cells that express the gene of interest, c-mpl, or the control EGFP gene. The occurrence of reconstitution in the implants of the irradiated SCID-hu animals was verified by the HLA Class I typing of the DNA derived from the cells of the colonies produced by the differentiation of CD34+ cells derived from the implants, ex vivo (Table 1). Progeny thymocytes produced by renewed thymopoiesis of these reconstituted CD34+ progenitor cells in vivo, were also HLA typed (Table 1). Thus the multi-lineage progeny cells of the donor CD34+ progenitor cells engrafted into the implants of the recipient SCID-hu animals possess the donor HLA Class I loci tissue types.

Levels of c-mpl or EGFP expression pre- and post-reconstitution of the CD34+ cells derived from the SCID-hu Thy/Liv implants. The untransduced CD34+ cells were negative for expression of either EGFP or c-mpl (Figure 1A). The transduced CD34+ cells that were reconstituted in the SCID-hu Thy/Liv implants showed a stable expression of c-mpl or EGFP gene (Figure 1B). Reconstitution of untransduced CD34+ cells expressed c-mpl at 24-28% in mock infection (absence of HIV-1) (Figures 1C and 1D). C-mpl and EGFP expression was maintained at 80-90% even at 9 weeks and up to 15 weeks post-reconstitution, 6 and 12 weeks post-infection, respectively (Figures 1C and 1D). Due to inherent limitations of the system, we were unable to obtain data beyond 15 weeks from the SCID-hu implants. Such limitations are the shrinking of the implant due to HIV-1 infection which causes eventual depletion of the thymocytes. When that happens, the implant "sack" containing the thymocytes and CD34+ cells becomes a hardened tissue from which it is difficult to tease out the single cell suspensions following the biopsies of the tissue of the human implants.

Table 1. Confirmation by HLA typing of reconstitution of the endogenous CD34+ cells of the irradiated SCID-hu Thy/Liv implants with exogenous human CD34+ cells. The primary implants (recipient tissue) following reconstitution of CD34+ cells were typed for HLA-A, -B, and –C loci by serology and low resolution DNA PCR at the UCSD Clinical Laboratories, San Diego, CA. After reconstitution, DNA was isolated from the cells of the colonies formed by the exogenous CD34+ cells and tissue typed for the HLA by DNA PCR. The donor and recipient CD34+ cells of the implants were also tissue typed for all the three HLA loci by serology and PCR, before CD34+ cell injection into the implants and thus prior to engraftment / reconstitution. Progeny thymocytes of the reconstituted CD34+ cells in the implants for HLA typing were derived from the reconstituted implants.

CD34+cells	Parent or progeny cell type	# Progeny colonies (C)/ implants (I) typed	*HLA Class I locus type*		
			A	B	Cw
Recipient implants	CD34+	N/A	34,68	39,52	07,16
Donor cells	CD34+	N/A	02,24	07,39	07,-
Reconstituted implants	Myeloid	12 (C)	02,24	07,39	07,-
	Erythroid	12 (C)	02,24	07,39	07,-
	Megakaryoid	6 (C)	02,24	07,39	07,-
	Thymocytes	12 (I)	02,24	07,39	07,-

The proviral loads of the thymocytes in the implants reconstituted with untransduced and EGFP/c-mpl-lentivirus transduced CD34+ cells were determined (Table 2A).

Expression of c-mpl (>80%) is not susceptible to HIV-1 mediated downregulation in the c-mpl- CD34+ cells transduced to express exogenous c-mpl following reconstitution (Table 2B). Partial re-acquirement of c-mpl expression occurs in untransduced and control EGFP-lentivirus transduced c-mpl- CD34+ cells, following functional reconstitution in the implants (Tables 2B and 2C), in concurrence with data of untransduced CD34+ cells in mock infection (Figures 1C and 1D).

Table 2A. HIV-1 proviral loads of the thymocytes derived from SCID-hu animal Thy/Liv implants following their reconstitution with lentiviral transduced human CD34+ cells. The proviral loads are of the HIV-1 infected thymocytes that coexisted with the untransduced or lentiviral transduced CD34+ cells in the human thymus/liver implants of the SCID-hu animals. The CD34+ cells are resistant to HIV-1 infection and were derived 6 wks post-reconstitution and at 3 wks post-infection of the implants / thymocytes. Standard deviations were calculated using CD34+ cells derived from implants of 4-6 animals.

CD34+ cell population that co-existed with the HIV-1 infected thymocytes in the Thy/Liv implants	Proviral loads in the thymocytes of the Thy/Liv implants: Number of HIV-1 NL4-3 copies / µg DNA
Untransduced c-mpl- CD34+ cells	3.2 ± 0.020x105
EGFP-lentivirus transduced c-mpl- CD34+ cells	3.4 ± 0.024x105
CMPL-lentivirus transduced CD34+ cells expressing exogenous c-mpl	3.7 ± 0.030x105

Table 2B. Percent expression of proteins in the untransduced and transduced human c-mpl- CD34+ cells derived from the Thy/Liv implants at 6 wks post-reconstitution and 3 wks post-infection. The expression of the CD34 antigen was determined by FACS analysis using anti-CD34-APC monoclonal antibody. EGFP expression was determined by its green color fluorescence. C-mpl expression was determined using an anti-c-mpl-PE monoclonal antibody. Standard deviations were calculated using CD34+ cells derived from implants of 4-6 animals. The CD34 antigen expression levels were similar for each group of animals whether they were mock or virus infected. The c-mpl expression values between the c-mpl and untransduced or EGFP transduced CD34+ control groups are significant ($p<0.05$).

Antigen or	CD34+ Cells (%)		EGFP Expressing CD34+ Cells (%)		C-mpl Expressing CD34+ Cells (%)	
Protein	Mock	HIV-1	Mock	HIV-1	Mock	HIV-1
CD34	95 ± 4	92 ± 8	98 ± 6	99 ± 8	92 ± 4	92 ± 6
EGFP	<1	<1	84 ± 5	87 ± 7	<1	<1
c-mpl	20 ± 3	9 ± 2	21 ± 3	10 ± 2	81 ± 5	85 ± 6

Table 2C. Functional reconstitution (CFU) of CD34+ cells following lentiviral transduction. Untransduced or lentiviral (EGFP or CMPL) transduced CD34+ cells derived from human fetal liver were reconstituted into the primary SCID-hu Thy/Liv implants. The CD34+ cells were then isolated from the reconstituted implants and the colonies formed in methylcellulose and megacult-C were counted, before reconstitution and 6 weeks after reconstitution. 500 input cells were seeded in each 35 mm petri dish containing a grid to facilitate colony counting. Standard deviations were calculated using CD34+ cells derived from implants of 4-6 animals. CFU of reconstituted animals were significantly different from those prior to reconstitution, $p<0.05$. CFU of the c-mpl transduced CD34+ cells was significantly higher than that of untransduced cells, $p<0.05$. EGFP transduced CD34+ cells whether reconstituted or not, exhibited a significantly lower CFU compared to the c-mpl transduced group, $p<0.05$.

	Myeloid Pre-/Post-CD34 Reconstitution		Erythroid Pre-/Post-CD34 Reconstitution		Megakaryocytoid Pre-/Post-CD34 Reconstitution	
Lentivirus transduction of CD34+ cells	Pre-	Post-	Pre-	Post-	Pre-	Post-
Untransduced	4 ± 2	32 ± 5	5 ± 3	33 ± 6	6 ± 3	41± 5
EGFP-transduced	2 ± 2	30 ± 5	4 ± 3	35 ± 5	5 ± 3	40 ± 6
c-mpl transduced	115 ± 8	121 ± 6	125 ± 7	132 ± 5	165 ± 6	169 ± 7

The re-acquirement of c-mpl expression in the HIV-1 infected animal implants following reconstitution was also inhibited in the untransduced or control EGFP-lentivirus transduced CD34+ cells (Table 2B). Whereas the mock infected implants expressed about 20% c-mpl, CD34+ cells from the virus-infected implants expressed 9-10% of c-mpl when analyzed by flow cytometry. However, in the c-mpl-lentivirus transduced CD34+ cells derived from mock and HIV-1 infected implants, both exhibit similar levels of c-mpl expression (>80%). This suggests that in these implants that were reconstituted with transduced c-mpl+ CD34+ cells, c-mpl expression was generally not susceptible to virus mediated down-regulation (Table 2B).

Knockdown of endogenous and exogenous c-mpl gene. In order to distinguish between any differences in functional contribution of endogenous and exogenous (ectopic) gene to levels of c-Mpl expression and CFU, we have performed the RNA interference (RNAi) of the c-mpl gene (Table 3 and Figure 2A). The causal effect of c-mpl on differentiation (CFU) of CD34+ progenitor cells was also confirmed using small interference RNA (siRNA) targeted towards c-mpl gene. The higher expression of exogenous c-mpl in transduced CD34+ cells significantly increases the CFU over and above that of endogenous c-mpl expression.

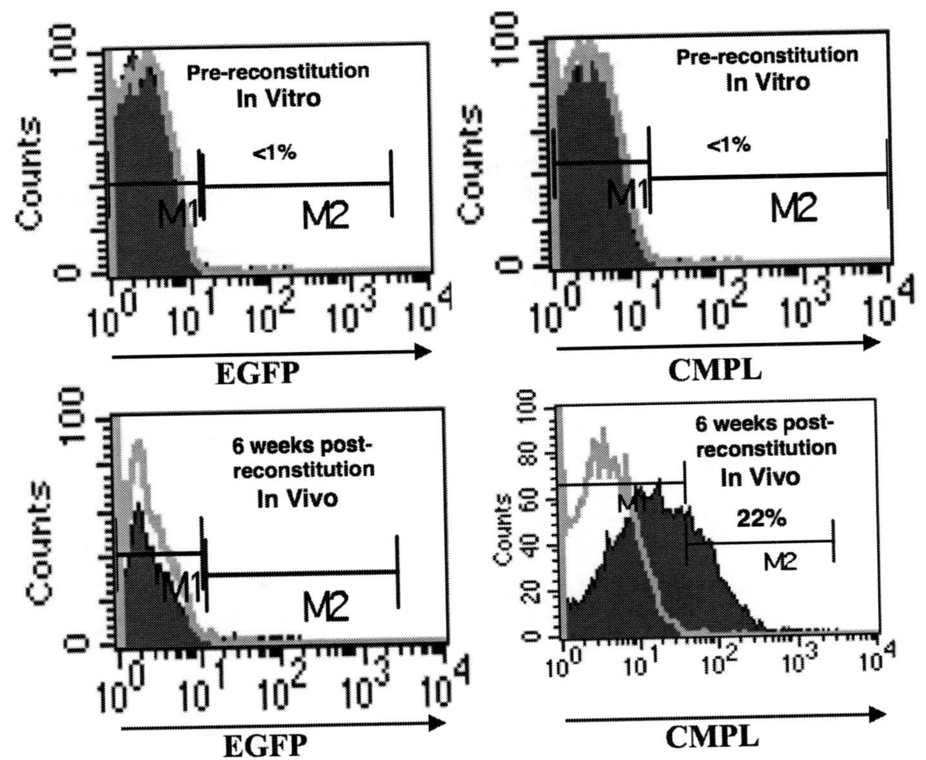

Figure 1A. Absence of EGFP or CMPL (c-mpl) expression in untransduced c-mpl- CD34+ cells. The green line represents the isotype control antibody staining of the untransduced CD34+ cells. FACS analyses were performed for EGFP fluorescence, or using anti-c-mpl-PE and anti-CD34-FITC monoclonal antibodies, for c-mpl expression. CD34 expression is not shown but cells were gated on CD34+ population to detect EGFP or c-mpl expression. M1 and M2 are the gates set in the FACS analyses to estimate the percent c-mpl or EGFP expression in the CD34+ cells. Analysis was performed using the control labeled isotype antibody stained in the absence of c-mpl primary antibody (M1), and in presence of c-mpl primary antibody or EGFP auto-fluorescence (M2). The green line represents isotype control staining of untransduced CD34+ cells. A representative set of histograms is shown here for illustration. Similar histograms were obtained with implants of the other sets of 4-6 animals.

Figure 1 continued on next page

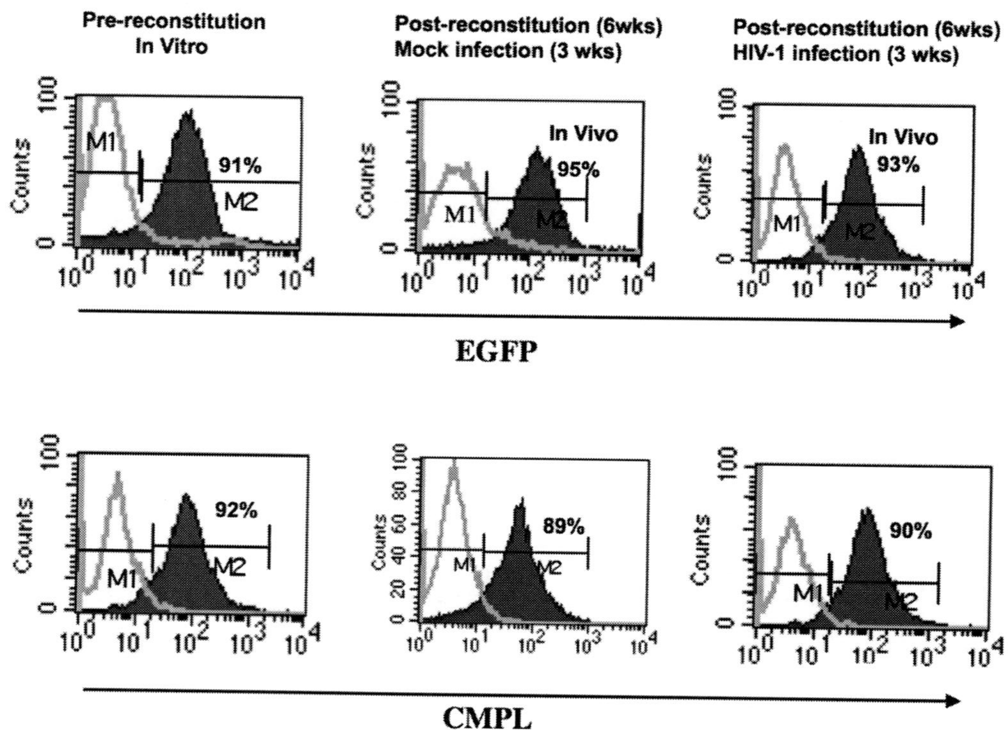

Figure 1B. Transduction of c-mpl- CD34+ cells with the control EGFP expressing lentivirus (Top Panels) and *c-mpl* gene expressing lentivirus (Bottom Panels). Top panels show a transduction efficiency of >90%, using EGFP fluorescence for the control lentivirus. Bottom panels show ~90% expression of c-mpl post-reconstitution, using anti-c-mpl-PE and anti-CD34-FITC monoclonal antibodies. Expression of c-mpl pre-reconstitution is 92%. CD34 expression is not shown but cells were gated on CD34+ population to detect EGFP or c-mpl expression. M1 and M2 are the gates set in the FACS analyses to estimate the percent c-mpl or EGFP expression in the CD34+ cells. Analysis was performed using the control isotype antibody stained in the absence of c-mpl primary antibody (M1), and in presence of c-mpl primary antibody or EGFP (M2). The green line represents isotype control staining of lentivirus transduced CD34+ cells. A representative set of histograms is shown here for illustration. Similar histograms were obtained with implants of the other sets of 4-6 animals.

Figure 1 continued on next page

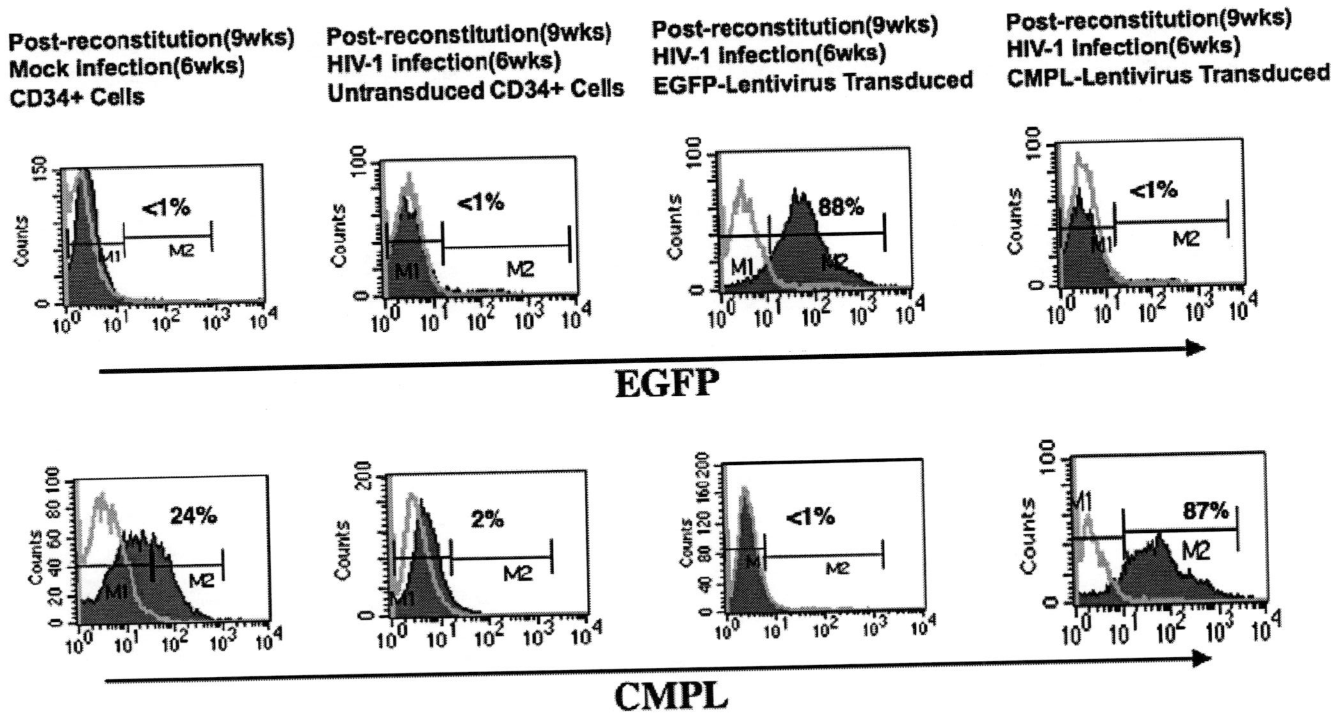

Figure 1C. Expression of EGFP and c-mpl following reconstitution of c-mpl- CD34+ cells at 9 weeks post-reconstitution and 6 weeks post-infection. Top third right histogram shows EGFP expression (88%) in the EGFP-lentivirus transduced CD34+ cells and the bottom right histogram shows c-mpl expression (87%). Untansduced CD34+ cells show 24% c-mpl expression post-reconstitution, in vivo. CD34 expression is not shown but cells were gated on CD34+ population to detect EGFP or c-mpl expression. M1 and M2 are the gates set in the FACS analyses to estimate the percent c-mpl or EGFP expression in the CD34+ cells. Analysis was performed using the control isotype antibody stained in the absence of c-mpl primary antibody (M1), and in presence of c-mpl primary antibody or EGFP (M2). The green line represents isotype control staining of untransduced or lentivirus transduced CD34+ cells as relevant. A representative set of histograms is shown here for illustration. Similar histograms were obtained with implants of the other sets of 4-6 animals.

Figure 1 continued on next page

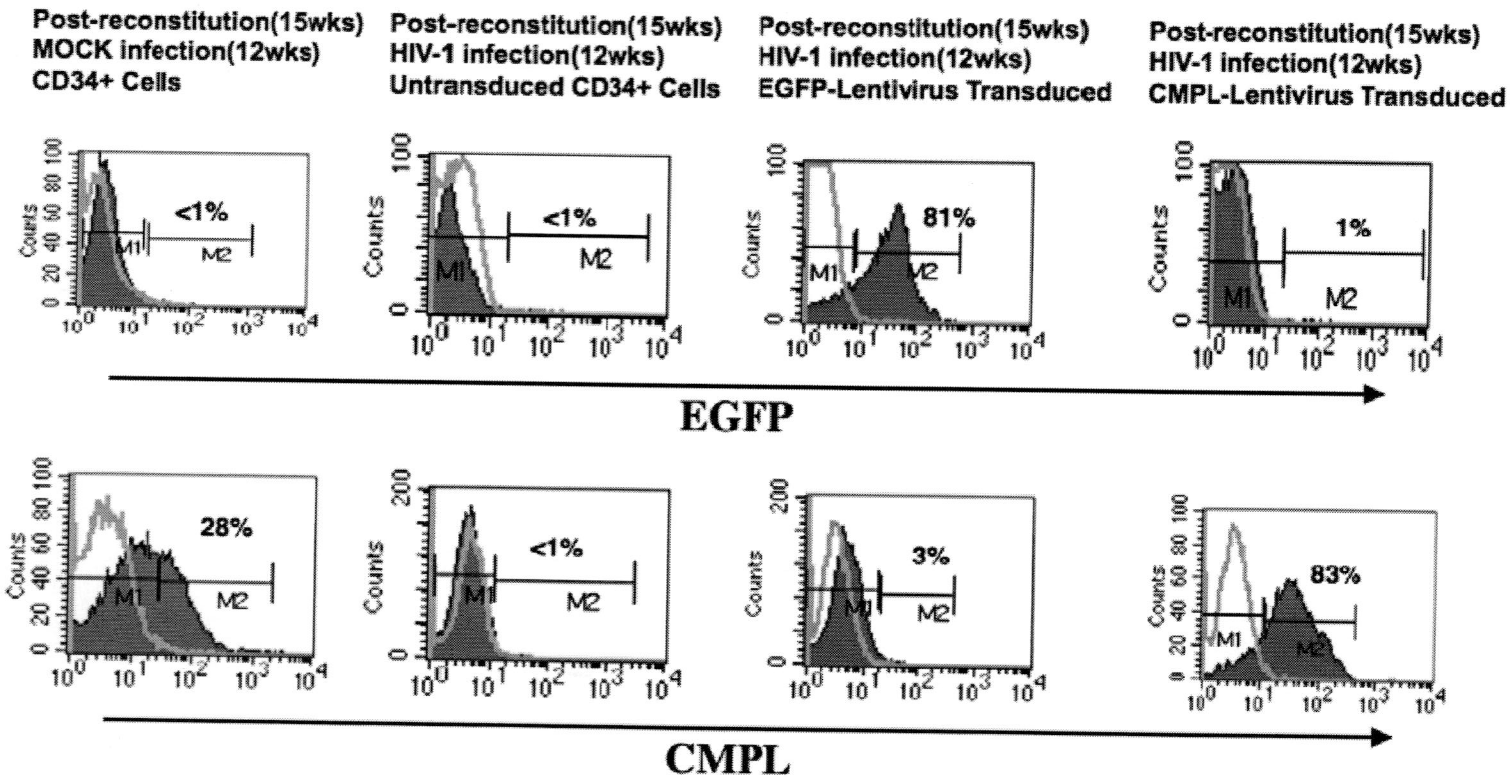

Figure 1D. Expression of EGFP and c-mpl following reconstitution of c-mpl- CD34+ cells at 15 weeks post-reconstitution and 12 weeks post-infection. Top third histogram show EGFP expression (81%) in the EGFP-lentivirus transduced CD34+ cells and the bottom right histogram shows c-mpl expression (83%). Untansduced CD34+ cells show 28% c-mpl expression post-reconstitution, in vivo. CD34 expression is not shown but cells were gated on CD34+ population to detect EGFP or c-mpl expression. M1 and M2 are the gates set in the FACS analyses to estimate the percent c-mpl or EGFP expression in the CD34+ cells. Analysis was performed using the control isotype antibody stained in the absence of c-mpl primary antibody (M1), and in presence of c-mpl primary antibody or EGFP (M2). The green line represents isotype control staining of untransduced or lentivirus transduced CD34+ cells as relevant. A representative set of histograms is shown here for illustration. Similar histograms were obtained with implants of the other sets of 4-6 animals.

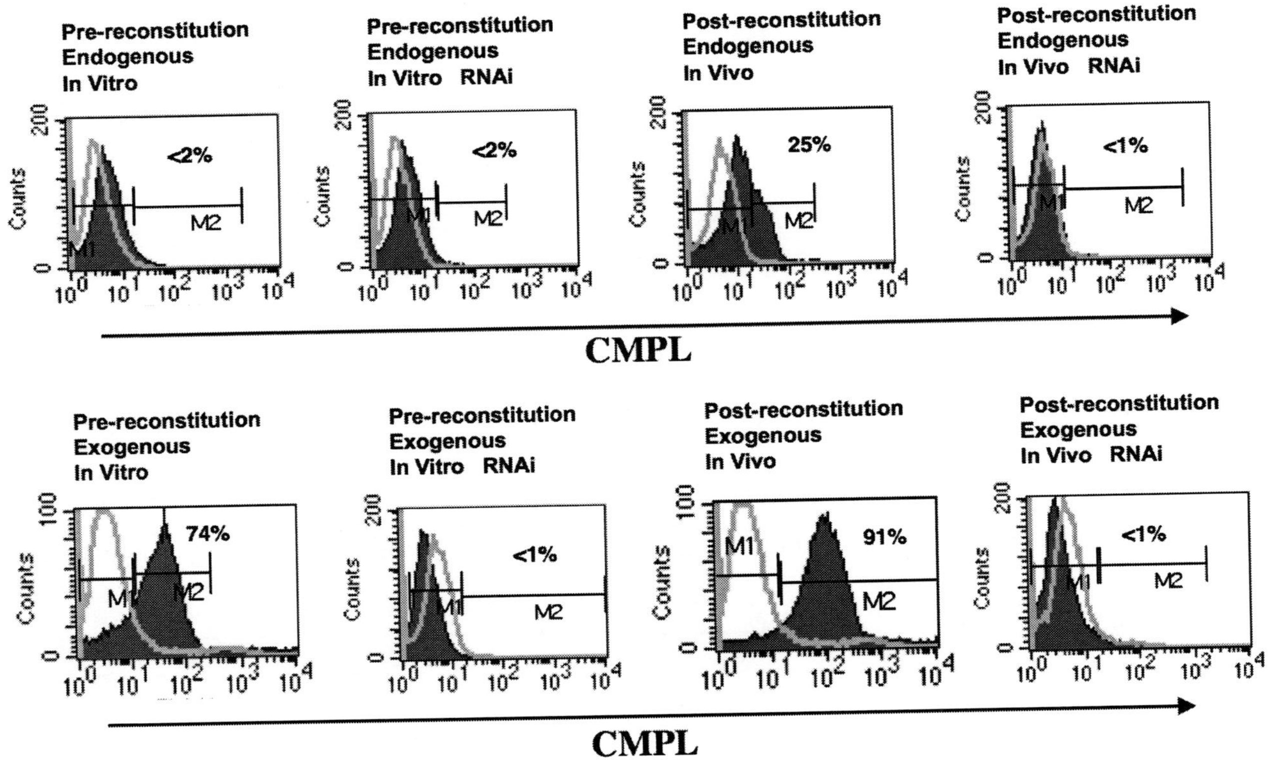

Figure 2. Knockdown (RNA interference, RNAi) of endogenous and exogenous c-mpl gene expression. Small interference RNA (siRNA) against the c-mpl gene was used. Both the endogenous and exogenous c-mpl expression in the untransduced (upper panels) and c-mpl transduced (lower panels) CD34+ cells, respectively, was knocked down post-reconstitution in vivo. The lentivirus carrying the siRNA against c-mpl gene was used to "super" transduce the lentivirus transduced c-mpl expressing CD34+ cells. Super transduction is super infection of the CD34+ cells with the siRNA lentivirus of the EGFP or c-mpl lentivirus infection. The siRNA was introduced into the CD34+ cells as described in the methods section prior to reconstitution in the SCID-hu implants. CD34 expression is not shown but cells were gated on CD34+ population to detect EGFP or c-mpl expression. M1 and M2 were the gates set in the FACS analyses to estimate the percent c-mpl or EGFP expression in the CD34+ cells. Analysis was performed using the control isotype antibody stained in the absence of c-mpl primary antibody (M1), and in presence of c-mpl primary antibody or EGFP (M2). The green line represents isotype control staining of transduced CD34+ cells. A representative set of histograms is shown here for illustration. Similar histograms were obtained with implants of the other sets of 4-6 animals.

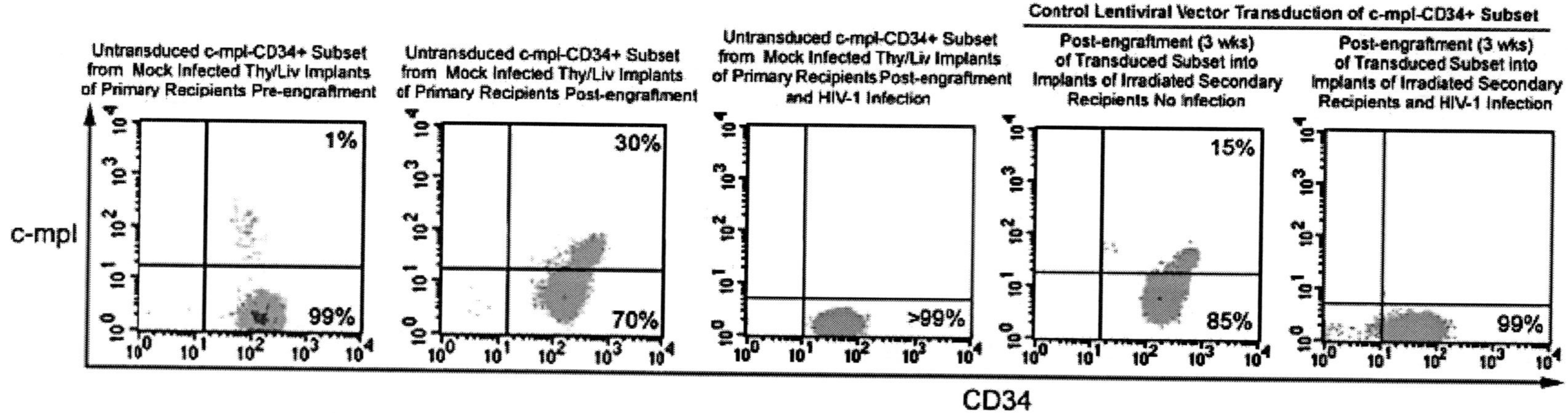

Figure 3A. Reacquirement of the c-mpl phenotype by the c-mpl- CD34+ subset cells, in the Thy/Liv implants of irradiated SCID-hu recipients. On the left histogram is the c-mpl- CD34+ cell subset from mock infected primary implants pre-engraftment. The 30% increase in c-mpl expression upon reconstitution is significant ($p<0.05$) (second histogram). HIV-1 infection aborts c-mpl expression from reacquirement (middle or third histogram). The levels of expression of the c-mpl post-reconstitution by the c-mpl- CD34+ cells transduced with the control EGFP-lentivirus are also shown (fourth histogram). The fifth histogram on the right represents control lentivirus vector transduced and reconstituted CD34+ cells wherein the implants were HIV-1 infected, but there was no c-mpl gene carried by the vector. CD34+ cells were gated and analyzed for c-mpl expression using anti-c-mpl-PE and anti-CD34-APC monoclonal antibodies. A representative set of histograms is shown here for illustration. Similar histograms were obtained with implants of the other sets of 4-6 animals.

Figure 3 continued on next page

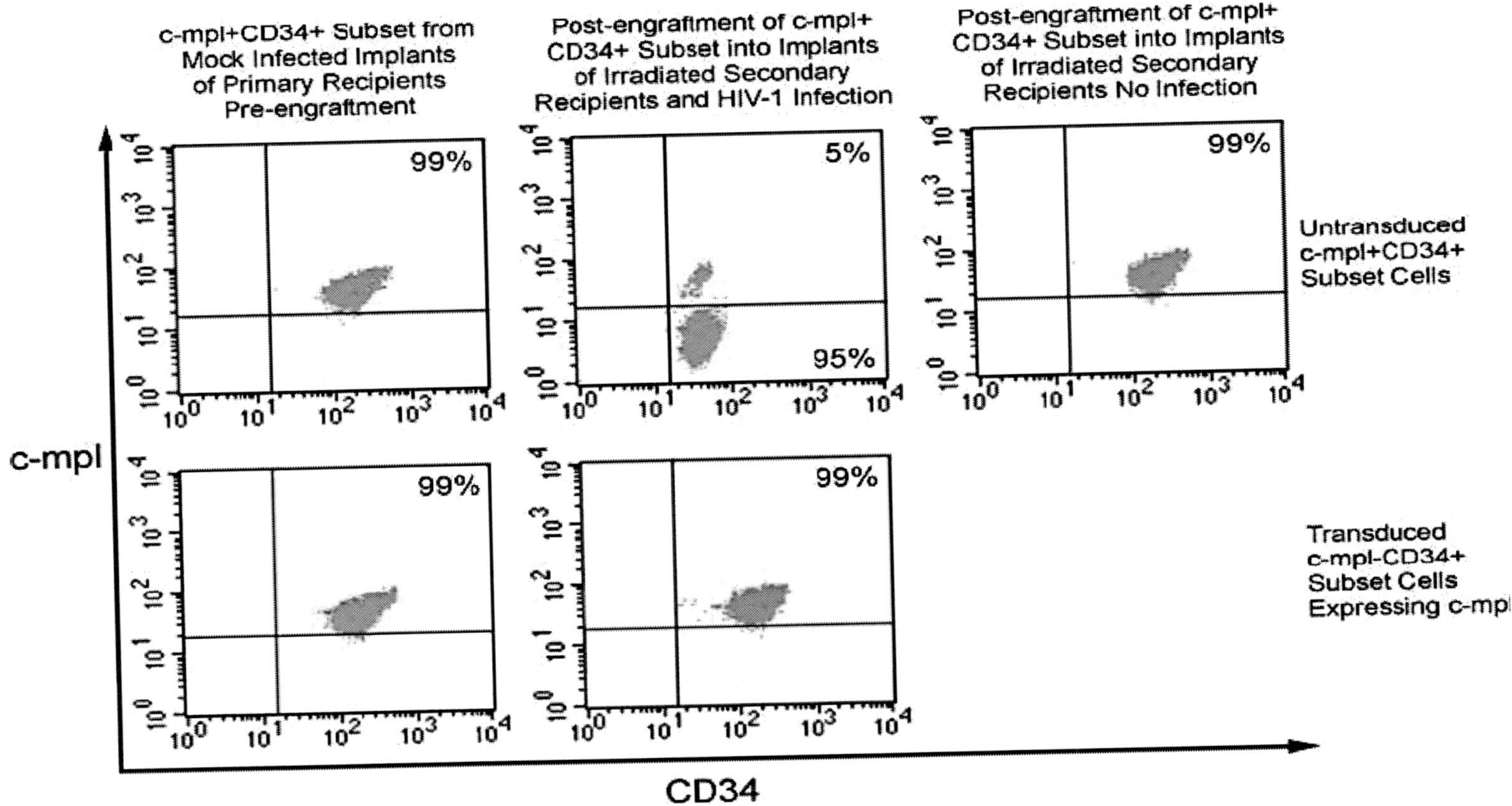

Figure 3B. Maintenance of c-mpl expression in lentivirus transduced c-mpl-CD34+ cells post-engraftment (12 weeks) and HIV-1 infection (9 weeks). The untransduced and c-mpl lentivirus transduced CD34+ cells were engrafted into a new stromal microenvironment of the Thy/Liv implants of irradiated SCID-hu recipients. The c-mpl- CD34+ cells transduced to express c-mpl, maintained the exogenous c-mpl expression during HIV-1 infection, whereas endogenous c-mpl expression in the was significantly reduced to 5% in the untransduced c-mpl+ CD34+ cells. Untransduced c-mpl+ CD34+ cells consisted of endogenous c-mpl which was susceptible to negative regulation by HIV-1 infection. Transduced c-mpl- CD34+ cells consisted of exogenous c-mpl expressed in the CD34+ cells through the lentivirus vector. CD34+ cells were gated and analyzed for c-mpl expression using anti-c-mpl-PE and anti-CD34-APC monoclonal antibodies.

Table 3. Functional activity (CFU) and c-Mpl expression of enodenous and exogenous c-mpl before and after gene knockdown. The siRNA was introduced into the CD34+ cells prior to reconstitution in the SCID-hu implants, as described in the methods section. The c-Mpl expression was determined by FACS analysis of the CD34+ cells using anti-c-mpl-PE monoclonal antibody. 500 input cells were seeded in each 35 mm petri dish containing a grid to facilitate colony counting. Standard deviations were calculated using CD34+ cells derived from implants of 4-6 animals.

Pre-/Post-Reconstitution	In Vitro/ In Vivo	Endogenous/ Exogenous	Intact/ Knockdown	Percent c-Mpl	CFU
Pre-Reconstitution	In Vitro	Endogenous	Intact	0±0	5±0
Pre-Reconstitution	In Vitro	Endogenous	Knockdown	0±0	0±0
Post-Reconstitution	In Vivo	Endogenous	Intact	24±3	140±8
Post-Reconstitution	In Vivo	Endogenous	Knockdown	3±0	12±2
Pre-Reconstitution	In Vitro	Exogenous	Intact	70±5	342±13
Pre-Reconstitution	In Vitro	Exogenous	Knockdown	2±0	9±1
Post-Reconstitution	In Vivo	Exogenous	Intact	90±6	441±15
Post-Reconstitution	In Vivo	Exogenous	Knockdown	5±0	19±3

Table 4. Rescue of hematopoiesis during HIV-1 infection *in vivo* as assessed by colony forming activity of the human CD34+ cells derived from the reconstituted implants. CFU of control untransduced c-mpl positive, control EGFP-lentivirus transduced c-mpl negative, and c-mpl-lentivirus transduced c-mpl negative CD34+ cells were determined. C-mpl-lentivirus transduced c-mpl negative CD34+ cells do express exogenous c-mpl which is not susceptible to down-regulation by HIV-1 infection. The untransduced c-mpl positive cells showed a drastic reduction in c-mpl expression which also reflected their loss of CFU, upon HIV-1 infection. CFU was assessed at 12 weeks post-engraftment / reconstitution and 9 weeks post-infection of the untransduced or lentivirus transduced CD34+ cells. 300 input cells were seeded. Standard deviations were calculated using CD34+ cells derived from implants of 4-6 animals

CD34 Subset	Transduction Status	Reconstitution Status	Implant Infection Status	% c-mpl	Colony Forming Activity		
					Myeloid	Erythroid	Megakaryoid
c-mpl+	Untransduced	Pre- reconstitution	No	95±4	89±8	84±7	101±10
c-mpl+	Untransduced	Post- reconstitution	No	92±5	87±6	81±7	98±9
c-mpl+	Untransduced	Post- reconstitution	Yes	5±2	6±3	5±2	2±2
c-mpl+	EGFP transduced	Pre-reconstitution	No	90±6	86±6	83±8	92±10
c-mpl+	EGFP transduced	Post-reconstitution	No	92±6	81±7	81±5	95±8
c-mpl+	EGFP transduced	Post-reconstitution	Yes	3±4	5±4	4±3	6±3
c-mpl-	Untransduced	Pre-reconstitution	No	3±2	2±2	3±2	4±3
c-mpl-	Untransduced	Post-reconstitution	No	19±3	19±5	17±5	21±4
c-mpl-	EGFP transduced	Pre- reconstitution	No	1±1	4±2	2±2	3±2
c-mpl-	EGFP transduced	Post- reconstitution	No	20±4	15±3	16±3	12±2
c-mpl-	c-mpl transduced	Pre- reconstitution	No	94±6	85±6	81±6	94±9
c-mpl-	c-mpl transduced	Post-reconstitution	No	92±5	86±7	80±8	92±9
c-mpl-	c-mpl Transduced	Post- reconstitution	Yes	90±8	89±5	86±6	97±7

Maintenance of c-mpl expression and CFU in lentivirus transduced c-mpl- CD34+ cells and rescue of hematopoiesis, during HIV-1 infection. Similar to the untransduced CD34+ cells, control (EGFP-lentivirus) vector transduced CD34+ cells show a partial re-acquirement of c-mpl expression upon reconstitution of the implants (Figures 3A). The c-mpl-lentivirus transduced CD34+ cells show a maximum recovery of c-mpl expression (~90%) at 12 weeks post-reconstitution and 9 weeks post-infection (Figure 3B, and Table 4). Reconstitution of the SCID-hu Thy/Liv implants with transduced CD34+ cells that express exogenous c-mpl showed about 90% rescue of multilineage hematopoiesis (Table 4). As expected, rescue did not occur in the reconstituted CD34+ cells that were transduced with the lentiviral vector carrying the control EGFP gene (Table 4).

Renewed thymopoiesis of exogenous CD34+ cells. Reconstitution with untransduced or EGFP-lentivirus transduced CD34+ cells yielded approximately 79-84% of CD4+CD8- thymocytes (Table 5). Implants reconstituted with c-mpl-lentivirus transduced CD34+ cells also attained maximal levels of single positive CD4+CD8- thymocytes (85%) compared to the double positive CD4+CD8+ thymocytes (11-16%), by 6 weeks post-reconstitution (Table

5). This confirms that renewed thymopoiesis is due to c-mpl expression. Hence this strategy shows promise for alleviation of cytopenias in HIV-1 infection.

Table 5. Generation of nascent single positive CD4+CD8- thymocytes upon reconstitution of the Thy/Liv implants with c-mpl-lentivirus transduced CD34+ cells. Renewed thymopoiesis occurs by 6 weeks post-reconstitution with untransduced and transduced CD34+ cells. Irradiation of the implants/animals prior to reconstitution depletes the preexisting human thymocytes. The thymocytes were analyzed by FACS using anti-CD4-FITC and anti-CD8-PE antibodies by gating on CD3+ cells using anti-CD3-PerCP antibody. Standard deviations were calculated using thymocytes derived from implants of 4-6 animals

	Reconstitution of Thy/Liv Implants with Untransduced or Lentivirus-Transduced CD34+ Cells					
Thymocyte Subset of the Thy/Liv Implants	Untransduced CD34: Percent Thymocytes		EGFP-lentivirus Transduced CD34: Percent Thymocytes		CMPL-lentivirus Transduced CD34: Percent Thymocytes	
	6 wks	12 wks	6 wks	12 wks	6 wks	12 wks
CD4+CD8-	81 ± 5	84 ± 3	79 ± 5	82 ± 4	83 ± 3	85 ± 3
CD8+CD4-	5 ± 1	4 ± 1	5 ± 1	6 ± 2	5 ± 1	4 ± 1
CD4+CD8+	14 ± 3	12 ± 2	16 ± 3	12 ± 2	12 ± 2	11 ± 2

Discussion

We have been able to confirm that following reconstitution, engrafted CD34+ cells produce multiple lineages of progeny including those of myeloid (granulocyte-macrophage), erythroid, megakaryocytoid, and thymocyte cell types, in SCID-hu Thy/Liv implants [28, 33]. These reconstituted CD34+ cells express the c-mpl transgene under the control of an exogenous promoter. The HLA Class I typing of the multiple progeny cells produced by the CD34+ progenitor cells of the reconstituted implants are an important testimony to the transgene being expressed in the progression of CD34+ cells towards multi-lineage differentiation. Renewed but transient multi-lineage hematopoiesis including thymopoiesis has been demonstrated in our previous reports [33]. Our new data show that we have been able to achieve a significant level of rescue of multilineage hematopoiesis despite HIV-1 infection.

HIV-1 influences c-mpl expression only when the latter's own endogenous promoter is present in the untransduced c-mpl+ CD34+ cells (Figure 3B). Also, the c-mpl expression is partially re-acquired by the c-mpl- CD34+ cells upon reconstitution when the SCID-hu Thy/Liv implants are not HIV-1 infected (Tables 2B and 2C; Figures 3A). Thus this process is reversible and even consistent with the transient revival of colony forming activity of the CD34+ cells when the SCID-hu animals were treated antiretroviral drugs [18]. It is well known that thrombopoietin (Tpo) is required for differentiation of CD34+ cells. Tpo is internalized by binding to its receptor c-Mpl, expressed on the surface of CD34+ cells. Tpo-stimulated cellular proliferation appears linked to receptor internalization, indicating that this process is essential for normal signal transduction. In spite of Tpo depletion, c-Mpl reappears on the cell surface, suggesting that c-Mpl recycling to the cell surface is not stimulated by Tpo [34]. However, in our SCID-hu implants, a reconstitution is likely to provide a stromal microenvironment that may enable the recycling to cell surface. Reconstitution may also trigger binding of the host transcription factors to the regulatory regions of the c-mpl gene, in vivo.

Increased c-mpl expression due to ectopic contribution in the transduced CD34+ cells enhances CFU commensurate with c-mpl expression (Figures 1C, 1D and 2A; Tables 2C, 3 and 4). This suggests that the ectopic c-mpl is also functionally active and that the CFU is proportional to c-Mpl expression. These data show that endogenous c-mpl expression of about 25-30% is increased to almost 85-90% due to ectopic c-mpl expression and the CFU is concomitant to c-mpl expression. That the knockdown of c-mpl expression and as a result the loss or reduction of CFU would occur due to RNA interference (RNAi), suggests accessibility of the c-mpl gene to siRNA directed against ectopic c-mpl as well which is expressed in the cellular cytoplasm.

When the c-mpl negative CD34+ cells are transduced with lentivirus to express c-mpl under the control of an exogenous housekeeping gene promoter, the c-mpl expression is not susceptible to the down-regulation effects of HIV-1 infection (Tables 2B and 4; Figure 3B). The regulation of c-mpl expression by HIV-1 infection has significant implications in that HIV-1 "influences" c-mpl expression which is involved in multi-lineage differentiation of CD34+ progenitor stem cells [20, 23, 35, 36]. The absence of c-mpl down-regulation in c-mpl lentivirus transduced CD34+ cells despite HIV-1 infection suggests potential effects by cellular factors/proteins on the regulation of endogenous c-mpl expression. The expression and function of c-mpl are presumably altered due to the indirect effects of virus infection of the thymocytes on the HIV-1 infection-resistant CD34+ cells present in the implants [15]. This is a topic for further and separate investigation wherein we will generate c-mpl promoter-reporter gene lentiviral DNA constructs for transduction of CD34+ cells and their reconstitution into implants. This will be done to establish regulatory mechanisms of c-mpl gene expression, in HIV-1 infection of the reconstituted implants. Secretion of cytokines in neural cells has been shown to occur due to interactions with the HIV-1 envelope protein, gp120, even in the absence of infection [18]. We have initiated investigation in this direction to determine how c-mpl gene expression under the control of its own "endogenous" promoter is regulated in HIV-1 infection, at the molecular and cellular levels.

After we placed the c-mpl gene under the control of a housekeeping gene promoter, susceptibility of its expression to the virus mediated indirect regulation seems to be significantly reduced or avoided. Since we had previously established a correlation between expression of c-mpl and CFU, we attempted to rescue hematopoiesis through stable c-mpl expression. In our previous transient renewal of hematopoiesis by antiretroviral drug therapy, the CFU declined by six weeks post infection after attaining a maximum at three weeks [18]. In our current study utilizing a gene therapeutic strategy, the CFU held steady even at six weeks post-infection (Table 2C). Technically it would not be feasible in this SCID-hu model system to maintain a sustained thymopoiesis since the newly generated progeny thymocytes are susceptible to de novo infection by the ever present HIV-1. The animal is not immune competent and hence a certain degree of immune responses to protect the host thymocytes as it occurs in humans is lacking, even though HIV infected patients also are immune compromised. Even if it were unable to derive significant benefits from renewed thymopoiesis due to pervasive HIV in the host human implant, still the approach is useful to alleviate hematopoietic inhibition of multiple lineages including thymocytes.

A concern with any transplant is the graft versus host disease (GVHD) but in this case a transfusion of purified CD34+ cells from a matched donor should not pose a serious conflict. Graft-versus-host-disease can largely be avoided by performing a T-cell depleted bone marrow transplant [37]. In addition, T-cells of umbilical cord blood have an inherent immunological immaturity [38], and unrelated donor transplants have a reduced incidence and severity of GVHD [39]. It has been shown that kidney transplants can be successfully performed in HIV-1 infected patients. A combination of HAART and immunosuppressant treatment ensured 70% renal graft survival for 2 years [40]. We believe that CD34+ cell engraftment as herein suggested is feasible in HIV-1 infected patients and that any potential adverse effects are manageable.

Despite the inducement of cytopenias by antiretroviral drug therapy (HAART), it can keep the HIV replication levels under control and in certain individuals, at non-detectable levels as estimated from proviral loads by PCR. We reported that aggressive HIV-1 replication increases hematopoietic inhibition in our SCID-hu model [18]. Moreover, long-term HAART in humans also induces cytopenias. It is expected that our preclinical translational research in vivo on CD34+ cell reconstitution therapeutic strategies may provide relief from cytopenias in HIV infected patients, eventually through bone marrow transplantation. Use of autologous CD34+ cells would be preferable but we have also discussed the feasibility of matched donor engraftments. Consequently, autologous bone marrow transplantation with transduced CD34+ cells expressing c-mpl may provide relief from hematopoietic abnormalities and ensuing cytopenias in HIV-infected patients.

Acknowledgments

This work was supported by NIH grant HL079846 to P.S.K. We thank Drs. Inder Verma and Mark Schmitt (The Salk Institute, La Jolla, CA) for providing the lentivirus vector.

References

[1] Mir, N., Costello, C., Luckit, J., and Lindley, R. 1989. HIV-disease and bone marrow changes: A study of 60 cases. *Eur. J. Hematol.* 42: 339-343.

[2] Sun N.C.J., Shapshack, P., Lachant, N.A., Hsu, M., Sieger, L., Schmid, P., Beall, G., and Imagawa, D.T. 1989. Bone marrow examination in patients with AIDS and AIDS-related complex. *Am. J. Clin. Pathol.* 92: 589-594.

[3] Miles, S.A., Lee, S., Hutlin, L., Zsebo, K.M., and Mitsuyasu, R.T. 1991. Potential use of Human stem cell factor as adjunctive therapy for Human immunodeficiency virus-related cytopenias. *Blood* 78: 3200-3208.

[4] Miles, S.A., Mitsuyasu, R.T., Moreno, J., Baldwin, G., Alton, N.K., Souza, L., and Glaspy, J.A. 1991. Combined therapy with recombinant granulocyte colony-

stimulating factor and erythropoietin decreases hematologic toxicity from zidovudine. *Blood* 77: 2109-2117.
[5] Utley, J.R. 1990. Pathophysiology of cardiopulmonary bypass: current issues. *J. Card. Surg.* 5: 177-189.
[6] Calenda, V., and Chermann, J.C. 1992. The effects of HIV on hematopoiesis. *Eur. J. Hematol.* 48: 181-186.
[7] Davis, B.R., and Zauli, G. 1995. Effect of human immunodeficiency virus infection on hematopoiesis. *Bailliers Clin. Hematol.* 8: 113-130.
[8] Geissler, R.G., Ottmann, O.G., Kleiner, K., Mentze, I.U., Bickelhaupt, A., Hoelzer, D., Ganser, A. 1993. Decreased hematopoietic colony growth in long-term bone marrow cultures of HIV-positive patients. *Res. Virol.* 144: 69-73.
[9] Re, M.C., Zauli, G., Furlini, G., Rarieri, S., Monari, P., Ramazzotti, E., and LaPlaca, M. 1993. The impaired number of circulating granulocyte / macrophage progenitors (CFU-GM) in human immunodeficiency virus type 1 infected subjects correlate with an active HIV-1 replication. *Arch. Virol.* 129: 53-64.
[10] Moses, A., Nelson, J., and Bagby Jr, G.C. 1998. The influence of human immunodeficiency virus-1 of hematopoiesis. *Blood* 91: 1479-1495.
[11] Chelucci, C., Casella, I., Federico, M., Testa, U., Macioce, G., Pelosi, E., Guerriero, R., Mariani, G., Giampaolo, A., Hasan, H.J., and Peschle, C. 1999. Lineage-specific expression of human immunodeficiency virus (HIV) receptor/coreceptors in differentiating hematopoietic precursors: Correlation with susceptibility to T- and M-tropic HIV and chemokine-mediated HIV resistance. *Blood* 94: 1590-1600.
[12] Ruiz, M.E., Ciala, C., Arthos, J., Kinter, A., Catanzaro, A.T., Adelsberger, J., Holmes, K.L., Cohen, O.J., and Fauci, A.S. 1998. Peripheral blood-derived CD34+ progenitor cells: CXC chemokine receptor 4 and CC chemokine receptor 5 expression and infection by HIV. *J. Immunol.* 161: 4169-4176.
[13] Shen, H., Cheng, T., Preffer, F.I., Dombkowski, D., Tomasson, M.H., Golan, D.E., Yang, O., Hofmann, W., Sodroski, J.G., Luster, A.D., and Scadden, D.T. 1999. Intrinsic Human immunodeficiency virus type 1 resistance of hematopoietic stem cells despite coreceptor expression. *J. Virol.* 73: 728-737.
[14] Sugira, K., Ovaizn, N., Pahwa, R., Kalyanaraman, V.S., and Pahwa, S. 1992. Effect of human immunodeficiency virus-1 envelope glycoprotein on in vitro hematopoiesis of umbilical cord blood. *Blood* 80: 1463-1469.
[15] Koka, P.S., Jamieson, B.D., Brooks, D.G., and Zack, J.A. 1999. Human immunodeficiency virus type-1 induced hematopoietic inhibition is independent of productive infection of progenitor cells in vivo. *J. Virol.* 73: 9089-9097.
[16] Zhang, J., Scadden, D.T., and Crumpacker, C.S. 2007. Primitive hematopoietic cells resist HIV-1 infection via p21. *J. Clin. Invest.* 117: 302-304.
[17] Jenkins, M., Hanley, M.B., Moreno, M.B., Wieder, E., and McCune, J.M. 1998. Human immunodeficiency virus-1 infection interrupts thymopoiesis and multilineage hematopoiesis in vivo. *Blood* 91: 2672-2678.
[18] Koka, P.S., Fraser, J.K., Bryson, Y., Bristol, G.C., Aldrovandi, G.M., Daar, E.S., and Zack, J.A. 1998. Human immunodeficiency virus type 1 inhibits multi-lineage hematopoiesis in vivo. *J. Virol.* 72: 5121-5127.
[19] Goncalves, F., Lacout, C., Villeval, J.L., Wendling, F., Vainchenker, W., Dumenil, D. 1997. Thrombopoetin does not induce lineage-restricted commitment of Mpl-R

expressing pluripotent progenitors but permits their complete erythroid and megakaryocytic differentiation. *Blood* 89: 3544-3553.

[20] Kaushansky, K. 1998. Thrombopoietin and the hematopoietic stem cell. *Blood* 92: 1-3.

[21] Kaushansky, K., Lin, N., Grossman, A., Humes, J., Sprugel, K.H., and Broudy, V.C. 1996. Thrombopoietin expands erythroid, granulocyte-macrophage, and megakaryocytic progenitor cells in normal and myelosuppressed mice. *Exp. Hematol.* 24: 265-269.

[22] Silvestris, F., Cafforio, P., Tucci, M., and Dammacco, F. 2002. Negative regulation of erythroblast maturation by Fas-L+/TRAIL+ highly malignant plasma cells: a major pathogenic mechanism of anemia in multiple myeloma. *Blood* 99: 1305-1313.

[23] Solar, G.P., Kerr, W.G., Zeigler, F.C., Hess, D., Donahue, C., De Sauvage, F.J., and Eaton, D.L. 1998. Role of c-mpl in early hematopoiesis. *Blood* 92: 4-10.

[24] Koka, P.S., Brooks, D.G., Razai, A., Kitchen, C.M., and Zack, J.A. 2003. HIV type 1 infection alters cytokine mRNA expression in thymus. *AIDS Res. Hum. Retr.* 19: 1-12.

[25] Sundell, I.B., and Koka, P.S. 2006. The SCID-hu mouse model as a stem cell host to recapitulate human hematopoiesis in HIV infection and serves as a tool for development of therapies for virus induced cytopenias. *J. Stem Cells* 1: 283-300.

[26] Louache, F., Henri, A., Bettaieb, A., Oksenhendler, E., Raguin, G., Tulliez, M., and Vainchenker, W. 1992. Role of human immunodeficiency virus replication in defective in vitro growth of hematopoietic progenitors. *Blood* 80: 2991-2999.

[27] Marandin, A., Katz, A., Oksenhendler, E., Tulliez, M., Picard, F., Vainchenker, W., and Louache, F. 1996. Loss of primitive hematopoietic progenitors in patients with human immunodeficiency virus infection. *Blood* 88: 4568-4578.

[28] Koka, P.S., Kitchen, C.M., and Reddy, S.T. 2004. Targeting c-Mpl for revival of human immunodeficiency virus type 1-induced hematopoietic inhibition when CD34+ progenitor cells are re-engrafted into a fresh stromal microenvironment in vivo. *J. Virol.* 78: 11385-11392.

[29] Soneoka, Y., Cannon, P.M., Ramsdale, E.E., Griffiths, J.C., Romano, G., Kingsman, S.M., and Kingsman, A.I. 1995. A transient three-plasmid expression system for the production of high titer retroviral vectors. *Nucl. Acid. Res.* 23: 628-633.

[30] Zufferey, R., Nagy, D., Mandel, R.J., Naldini, L., and Trono, D. 1997. Multiply attenuated lentiviral vector achieves efficient gene delivery in vivo. *Nat. Biotechnol.* 15: 871-875.

[31] Burns, J.C., Friedman, T., Driever, W., Burrascano, M., and Yee J-K. 1993. Vesicular stomatitis virus G glycoprotein pseudotyped retroviral vectors: concentration to very high titer and efficient gene transfer into mammalian and nonmammalian cells. *Proc. Natl. Acad. Sci. USA.* 90: 8033-8037.

[32] Vignon, I., Mornon, J-P., Cocault, L., Mitiavila, M-T., Tambourin, P., Gisselbrecht, S., and Souyri, M. 1992. Molecular cloning and characterization of MPL, the human homolog of the v-mpl oncogene: Identification of a member of the hematopoietic growth factor receptor superfamily. *Proc. Natl. Acad. Sci. USA.* 89: 5640-5644.

[33] Withers-Ward, E.S., Amado, R.G., Koka, P.S., Jamieson, B.D., Kaplan, A.H., Chen, I.S.Y., and Zack, J.A. 1997. Transient renewal of thymopoiesis in HIV infected human thymic implants following antiviral therapy. *Nat. Med.* 3: 1102-1109.

[34] Dahlen, D.D., Broudy, V.C., and Drachman, J.G. 2003. Internalization of the thrombopoietin receptor is regulated by 2 cytoplasmic motifs. *Blood* 102: 102-108.

[35] Rasko, J.E., O'Flaherty, E., and Begley, C.G. 1997. Mpl ligand (MGDF) alone and in combination with SCF promotes proliferation and survival of human megakaryocyte, erythroid and granulocyte/macrophage progenitors. *Stem Cells* 15: 33-42.

[36] Yoshida, M., Tsuji, K., Ebihara, Y., Muraoka, K., Tanaka, R., Miyazaki, H., and Nakahata, T. 1997. Thrombopoietin alone stimulates the early proliferation and survival of human erythroid, myeloid aand multipotential progenitors in serum-free culture. *Br. J. Hematol.* 98: 254-264.

[37] Morishima, Y., Sasazuki, T., and Inoko, H. 2002. The clinical significance of human leukocyte antigen (HLA) allele compatibility in patients receiving a marrow transplant from serologically HLA-A, HLA-B, and HLA-DR matched unrelated donors. *Blood* 99: 4200-4206.

[38] Grewal, S.S., Barker, J.N., Davies, S.M., and Wagner, J.E. 2003. Unrelated donor hematopoietic cell transplantation: marrow or umbilical cord blood? *Blood* 101: 4233-4244.

[39] Laughlin, M.J., Barker, J., and Bambach, B. 2001. Hematopoietic engraftment and survival in adult recipients of umbilical-cord blood from unrelated donors. *N. Engl. J. Med.* 344: 1815-1822.

[40] Kumar, M.S., Sierka, D.R., Damask, A.M., Fyfe, B., McAlack, R.F., Heifets, M., Moritz, M.J., Alvarez, D., and Kumar, A. 2005. Safety and success of kidney transplantation and concomitant immunosuppression in HIV-positive patients. *Kidney Intl.* 67: 1622-1629.

In: Stem Cell Therapy and Uses in Medical Treatment
Editor: Prasad S. Koka, pp. 143-157
ISBN: 978-1-61324-008-3

Chapter 9

Neurotrophin in Obstetrics and Gynaecology

Chinmoy K. Bose*
Institut für Reproduktionsmedizin
Domagkstraße 11
48149 Münster, Germany

Abstract

Since Rita Levi Montalcini and Stanley Cohen received Nobel Prize for their pioneering work on nerve growth factor (NGF), its role in female reproductive system has been reinforced in last two decades. The neurotrophins (NT) including nerve growth factor (NGF) are a family of related growth factors and their respective receptor tyrosine kinases that are of major importance in the regulation of neuronal survival and differentiation. While role of NGF in mast cell-mediated egg implantation and inhibition of rejection were primary concern at their time, in the ovary NGF can help in the differentiation process by which ovarian follicles become responsive to gonadotrophins. They help in follicular maturation, steroid secretion and ovulation in the ovary, by inducing the FSH receptor (FSHR). Due to the pleiotropism, NGF is mandatory for the success of pregnancy, while progesterone helping to maintain local levels of NGF in utero. In endometriosisi and polycystic ovarian disease it has major role to play. An autocrine role of NGF in breast cancer and epithelial ovarian cancer (EOC) is evident now. Thus its study will infuse new insight in diseases of both obstetrics and gynaecology.

Keywords: Nerve growth factor, uterus, ovary, endomtrium, placenta, decidua, breast.

* Address for correspondence: Dr Chinmoy K Bose, 8D, Mathur Sen Garden Lane, Kolkata 700006, India. Email: ckbose@hotmail.com; Fax: 00913328430741

Introduction

In 1951, selective growth stimulating effects of mouse sarcoma on the sensory and sympathetic nervous system of the chick embryo paved the way for materializing the nerve growth-stimulating factor (Levi-Montalcini and Hamburger 1951). The Nerve Growth Factor (NGF) was officially established in 1964 by an article in single authorship of Professor Levi-Montalcini in the annals of New York academy of Science (Levi-Montalcini 1964).

Gradually neurotrophins (NTs), which include NGF and many like proteins and their receptors, came into existence. Tremendous ramification of the subject is palpable by nearly 30000 pubmed entries till date. Neurotrophins induce the survival of neurons signaling particular cells to survive, differentiate, or grow within both the central and peripheral nervous system. Neurotrophic factors are secreted by target tissue. They prevent the associated neuron from initiating programmed cell death. Neurons then can survive by target-derived trophic action of this factor. Four structurally related factors are nerve growth factor (NGF), brain-derived neurotrophic factor (BDNF), neurotrophin-3 (NT-3), and neurotrophin-4 (NT-4). Another novel neurotrophin-1 (NNT1), structurally unrelated to NGF, BDNF, NT-3 and NT-4 is also described. Among receptors, p75 is a low affinity neurotrophin receptor, to which all neurotrophins bind. It is a member of the tumour necrosis super family. The Tyrosine kinases receptors, Trk family include TrkA, TrkB, and TrkC, and will only bind with specific neurotrophins, but with a much higher affinity.

As for its significance in reproductive system Professor Levi-Montalcini herself visualized that NGF could participate in fertilization mechanisms by cytoskeletal-mediated activation of spermatozoa locomotion much in the same way as in neurite outgrowth, or by favoring egg implantation, via inhibition of rejection through the immune system. The latter hypothesis was assessed seeing the effect of NGF on uterine mast cells, which, through histamine release, are postulated to initiate the local immune reaction (Beer *et al* 1984). Though female reproductive system was not touched in this respect, relevance of this subject has not only been updated over all the years but newer developments and hypotheses have made it really a vast field. which now very well includes it.

Romantic Love

Emanuele *et al* (2006) examined whether the early romantic phase of a loving relationship bears any relationship with changes in circulating levels of NTs. Plasma levels of NGF, BDNF, NT-3 and NT-4 were measured in subjects who had recently fallen in love and compared with those of two control groups, consisting of subjects who were either single or were already engaged in a long-lasting relationship. NGF level was significantly higher in the subjects in love. They opined that raised NGF levels in the bloodstream might lead to some behavioural and/or psychological features associated with falling in love.

Ovary

Mouse sarcoma was the first detected source of NGF. Snake venom, which was primarily used for its degrading enzyme, phosphodiesterase to degrade the nucleic acid of sarcoma fraction, accidentally proved to be having lot of NGF in it. However, NGF was detected first not in female but in male reproductive system. As Rita Levi-Montalcini showed in her Nobel lecture, NGF's role in spermatozoa locomotion much in the same way as in neurite outgrowth, NGF-like immunoreactivity was found in guinea pig (Chapman *et al* 1979, Harper *et al* 1979) and rabbit prostate, and in bull semen and seminal vesicle. Furthermore, in the mouse testis, immunoreactivity was shown to be present in germ cells, and a possible role for NGF in sperm maturation or motility was hypothesized (Ayer-LeLievre *et al* 1988).

Differences in NGF concentrations between men and women (in both phases of the menstrual cycles) are statistically significant (Martocchia *et al* 2002). We now know that the difference of serum NGF concentrations between the follicular and luteal phase in each woman is also statistically significant. A Japanese group first showed effect of NGF on ovary in as early as 1970 (Akasu *et al* 1970). But, Ojeda and his groups vastly study regulation of ovarian function over last four decades. However, they could start relate the subject with NGF in as late as 1990.

Treatment of neonatal rats with antibodies to nerve growth factor (NGF Ab) resulted in failure of the sympathetic (noradrenergic and neuropeptide-Y) nerves to develop (Lara *et al* 1990). Cross-linking of [^{125}I] NGF to ovarian membranes followed by immunoprecipitation, sodium dodecyl sulfate-polyacrylamide gel electrophoresis, and autoradiography showed the presence of an approximately 90-kilodalton molecular species, which corresponds in size to the predominant NGF receptor species, cross-linked to its ligand (Dissen *et al* 1990). Ovarian NGF receptors may be of neuronal origin and reach the gland exclusively by anterograde axonal transport. RNA blot hybridization demonstrated that the ovary expresses NGF receptors mRNA species that encodes p75NTR and, thus, implicated the ovary itself as a site of NGF receptors synthesis. NGF receptors mRNA levels decreased abruptly after the first ovulation, suggesting that NGF receptors may be synthesized in growing follicles and that this capacity is lost after follicular rupture and luteinization.

NGF and NT-3, two members of the neurotrophin family, was then identified in the rat ovary and one of its receptors (p75NTR) had been localized to the innervation and thecal cells of developing follicles. Although NGF supports the sympathetic innervation of the gland, the extent to which follicles are innervated appears to be defined by the differential expression of NGF receptors in the theca of developing follicles. The presence of NGF receptors in steroid-producing cells suggests a direct involvement of neurotrophins in the regulation of gonadal endocrine function (Ojeda *et al* 1992). The mature mammalian ovary has now been shown to synthesize several neurotrophins, including NGF, NT-3, and NT-4/5. The ovary also expresses some of the neurotrophin receptors, including p75NTR, trkB (the receptor for NT-4/5 and BDNF) and trkA (the NGF receptor) (Dissen *et al* 1995).

Primate ovary contains an intrinsic network of neuron-like cells (Dissen *et al* 1996). Because such an intrinsic neuronal network has not been detected in rodents or other non-primate species, it would appear that its presence in the primate ovary might have evolutionary significance. Gap junctions functionally couples thecal cells of Graafian follicles, and the ovulatory rupture requires dissociation of thecal cell-cell communication,

NGF-induced activation of trkA receptors in isolated ovarian thecal cells disrupts cell to cell communication by affecting the functional integrity of gap junctions. Thus, cell-specific activation of trkA receptors in periovulatory follicles may provide one of the signals involved in inducing the cellular dissociation of the follicular wall that precedes ovulatory rupture (Mayerhofer *et al* 1996).

Formation and development of mammalian follicles requires the concerted action of genes originally thought to be only involved in cell differentiation/survival of neuronal cells, and genes that may control the growth, differentiation, and cell-cell interactions of somatic and germ cells in the ovary (Ojeda *et al* 2000). Presence of these intrinsic neurons in the human ovary, similar to those previously found in other species, proved that they might be engaged in regulating common, phylogenetically conserved, ovarian functions. It also raised the possibility that their dysfunction may contribute to the manifestation of particular ovarian pathologies (Anesetti *et al* 2001).

The growth of primordial follicles is retarded in the absence of NGF, indicating that NGF contributes to facilitating early follicular development. One of the functions of NGF in the developing ovary is to facilitate the differentiation process by which early growing follicles become gonadotropin-dependent during postnatal life, and it does so by increasing the synthesis of FSHRs (Romero *et al* 2002).

Implantation

Immunoreactions for NGF, TrkA and p75NTR were also detectable in epithelial cells and muscle cells of the ampulla and isthmus of the oviduct, and in epithelial cells and uterine glands of the uterus. These results strongly suggest autocrine and paracrine regulation of reproductive function by NGF in the reproductive tract (Ren *et al* 2005). Long back, isolation of human NGF from placental tissue by using the chicken embryo dorsal root ganglia assay showed highest levels of NGF activity in placental cotyledons amongst amnion, placental cotyledons, cord serum, fetal serum, and maternal serum (Goldstein *et al* 1978). Eventually large-scale isolation of human NGF of placental origin, and its immunological characterization was possible in 1990 (Bigon *et al* 1990). Using reverse transcriptase-polymerase chain reaction (RT-PCR), trophoblast, amnion/chorion and maternal decidua showed the expression of NGF mRNA both in early gestation and at term. By immunohistochemistry, the immunoreactive NGF was found in the cyto and syncytial trophoblast cells, chorionic mesodermal cells. Vessel endothelial cells were stained in maternal compartments, while fetal vessels were unstained. Thus, human placenta is a potent neuroendocrine organ throughout gestation (Toti *et al* 2006).

Stress and substance P (SP) injection significantly increased the abortion rate and up-regulated decidual NGF and TrkA expression compared with the control. Stress, elicited by environmental and social conditions, is known to affect the homeostasis of the nervous, endocrine and immune systems. In pregnancy, perceived stress results in a predomination of inflammatory abortion-associated Th1 (helper T cell 1) cytokines over immunosuppressive, pregnancy-protective-associated Th2 cytokines, putatively via neuropeptide substance P (SP). NGF being an important trophic factor for sympathetic neurons has been implicated in the responsiveness of immune-competent cells through its functional receptor, TrkA. NGF enhances local mast cell number in decidua proving a cross talk with nerve in decidualisation. Dendritic cell expressing trkA and p75NTR may have some role to play through inflammation. Monocyte and resultant macrophages may also act in this pathway (Tometten *et al* 2004).

NGFβ acts as a proximal mediator in the hierarchical network of immune rejection by mediating an abortogenic environment comprised of classical signs of neurogenic inflammation (Tometten *et al* 2006). NGF is also mandatory for the success of pregnancy via inhibition of paternal major histocompatibilty antigen, MHC II molecule expression on trophoblast cells. This is supported by published evidence on progesterone, the hormone of pregnancy, which maintains local levels of NGF (Tometten *et al* 2005).

Pregnancy

In the pregnant uterus, a pronounced transient decrease of autonomous innervation evidenced by a marked axonal degeneration of myometrial and perivascular adrenergic fibers has been reported in animal models and in humans. However, several factors have been implicated in the pregnancy-related uterine denervation: 1) the mechanical stretch induced by the growing fetus 2) the high levels of circulating ovarian steroids during pregnancy and 3) a dilution of neurotrophic factors in the pregnant uterus. The density of sympathetic innervation in effector organs is directly correlated to the expression of neurotrophins especially NGFß. But previous studies have analyzed the presence and fluctuations of NGFß in the pregnant uterus with conflicting results (Lobos *et al* 2005).

The physiological denervation occurring in the uterus and uterine artery during pregnancy is related to a decrease in the availability of NGF by nerve fibers, and to the impossibility to mediate its effect due to a remarkable decrease in the signal-transducing TrkA receptor (Naves *et al* 1998). In all the uterine regions analysed, NGF-protein levels showed a decline at term pregnancy, but in no case was this change statistically significant. After delivery, NGF-protein levels showed a marked increase in the cervix as well as in both the fertile and empty horns. So it was thought that alterations in NGF-protein do not account for the impairment of uterine sympathetic innervation during pregnancy, but may contribute to their recovery after delivery (Brauer *et al* 2000, Varol *et al* 2000).

To solve this dilemma NGF metabolism was carefully scrutinized. It was seen that NGF is synthesized as a precursor protein (proNGF) that is processed posttranslationally into mature 13.5-kDa NGF-ß. The processing of proNGF results also in a series of high-molecular-weight intermediate forms whose biological roles are not well understood. High-molecular weight glycosylated proNGF forms have been detected in a wide variety of cells in vitro and in vivo. ProNGF forms and not mature NGF-ß are the predominant forms in human and rat brains and several peripheral tissues. ProNGF and its proteolytically processed protein products may differentially activate pro- and antiapoptotic cellular responses through preferential activation of TrkA or p75NTR. Therefore, it was suggested that the balance between cell death and survival may be determined by the ratio of secreted proNGF and mature NGF-ß (Chao and Bothwell 2000).

Alterations in NGF isoforms during pregnancy, accumulation of proNGF, and decreased ratios of mature NGF-ß to proNGF in the pregnant rat uterus coinciding with the transient uterine axonal degeneration of the pregnant myometrium then corroborated the results reported by previous studies. Under certain circumstances when the balance between a proneurotrophin and mature neurotrophin favors the proneurotrophins, it may cause degeneration of neurons (Krizsan-Agbas *et al* 2000) and this happens in pregnant uterus.

It is worthwhile to discuss hormonal influence on such denervation. Sympathetic innervation of the adult rodent uterus undergoes cyclic remodelling. Terminal sympathetic axons degenerate when estrogen levels rise and regenerate when estrogen levels decline. Reduced NGF or NT-3 is not responsible for the estrogen-induced denervation. Estrogen also raised BDNF protein and mRNA in myometrium and endometrium (Krizsan-Agbas *et al* 2000). Estrogen alters neuritogenic properties of uterus by regulating BDNF synthesis, which inhibits sympathetic neurite outgrowth.

The human cervix in nonpregnant, early pregnant and term pregnant women was by far more densely innervated than the rest of the uterus. No obvious difference in nerve density was observed between nonpregnant, early pregnant and term pregnant women, and still during labor the innervation appeared morphologically preserved. It is suggested that the segmental difference in innervation of the human uterus (corpus versus cervix) may have specific importance for myometrial and cervical contractility during pregnancy and parturition (Bryman *et al* 1987). Women display markedly decreased BDNF serum levels before and after childbirth. This phenomenon might reflect an increased risk for the development of mood disorders in the perinatal period. However, the individual serum concentration of BDNF alone did not predict maternal depression (Lommatzsch *et al* 2006).

The presence of biologically active NGF in the peripheral circulation of women during pregnancy, labour and lactation was investigated. Using a sensitive immunoenzymatic assay (ELISA), an approximately five-fold increase in plasma NGF levels was found during labour and lactation compared with the concentrations found at the term of gestation or in control healthy women (Luppi *et al* 1993). Since labour and lactation are characterized by activation of the hypothalamo-pituitary-adrenal axis and by high plasma levels of the neurohypophyseal hormone oxytocin, and since the intravenous injection of oxytocin in female rats causes a 176% increase in the hypothalamic levels of NGF, it is possible that the increased amount of circulating NGF is correlated with one or both of these events.

Intrauterine Growth Restriction

Circulating NGF, BDNF, NT-3 and NT-4 levels in IUGR and appropriate for gestational age (AGA) full term fetuses and neonates (day-1 [N1] and day-4 [N4]) and in their mothers was measured. While no statistically significant differences existed between IUGR and AGA maternal, fetal and neonatal levels of BDNF, NT-3 and NT-4, NGF was significantly higher in AGA than IUGR maternal (p=0.007), fetal (p=0.01), neonatal day 1 (p=0.043) and 4 (p=0.003) plasma. NGF positively correlated with the infants' centiles and birthweights proving brain sparing effect of BDNF, NT-3 and NT-4, in contrast to NGF levels, which are higher in the AGA group (Malamitsi-Puchner *et al* 2007).

S100B, a neural protein found in high concentrations after cell injury in the nervous system, is increased in serum of women whose pregnancies are complicated by IUGR and whose newborns develop IVH (Gazzolo *et al* 2006). Some pathological conditions that develop during pregnancy and are related to hypoxic stress can affect the elevation of S100B concentration in the amnion (Tskitishvili *et al* 2006). Over expression of S100B results in enhanced cell survival under stress conditions, increased cell proliferation, a reduced extent of apoptosis, and decreased responsiveness to the differentiating effect of NGF to the benefit of condition prevailing in IUGR (Arcuri *et al* 2005).

Endometriosis

Possible role for nerve growth factor (NGF) in the mechanism of pain and hyperalgesia induced by deep adenomyotic nodules and other forms of endometriosis was investigated. It was hoped that this might clarify the relationship between endometriotic lesions and the surrounding nerves also (Anaf *et al* 2002). Immunohistochemistry with antibodies against NGF, NGF specific tyrosine-kinase receptor (Trk-A) and S-100B protein was performed in endometriotic lesions. NGF expression was significantly stronger in deep adenomyotic nodules (DAN) than in ovarian (OE) and peritoneal endometriosis (PE), both in the proliferative phase in the glands and in the stroma. NGF expression in DAN is also significantly stronger than in OE and PE in the secretory phase in the glands and in the stroma. Perineurial and intraneurial invasion by endometriotic lesions were found only in deep adenomyotic nodules and not in the other forms of endometriosis. The specific receptor for NGF (Trk-A) is expressed in all the nerves that were included in the biopsies. The strong expression of the NGF-TrkA pathway in deep adenomyotic nodules could explain why this type of lesion infiltrates in richly innervated anatomical sites. Thus it is proposed that NGF may normally regulate the differentiation of the mesenchyme into uterine myocytes through paracrine mechanisms and that an early disturbance of this process plays a key role in the subsequent development of adenomyosis (Green *et al* 2003).

Tamoxifen can upregulate *NGF* gene that in turn may be responsible for the development of adenomyosis. Increased adenomyosis incidence and severity was evident in the tamoxifen-treated mice with increasing age. Pathological examination of uterine tissues showed there to be extensive down-growth of endometrial glands and stroma into thickened, abnormal myometrium that had disorganised fascicles of smooth muscle and increased interstitial collagen deposition Results provide a basis for understanding the mechanism for tamoxifen induced tissue remodelling and the development of adenomyosis (Green *et al* 2001).

In an experiment to investigate the topographical relationship between nerve fibers and peritoneal endometriotic lesions and to determine the origin of endometriosis-associated nerve fibers in a retrospective nonrandomized study, was done. The endometriosis-associated nerve fibers are accompanied by immature blood vessels within the stroma. Endometriotic cells express NGF and NT-3. Growth-associated protein 43, a marker of neural outgrowth and regeneration, is expressed in endometriosis-associated nerve fibers but not in existing peritoneal nerves. The data provide the first evidence of direct contact between sensory nerve fibers and peritoneal endometriotic lesions. This implies that the nerve fibers play an important role in the etiology of endometriosis-associated pelvic pain (Mechsner *et al* 2007). Moreover, emerging evidence suggests that peritoneal endometriotic cells exhibit neurotrophic properties.

Nerve growth factor and nerve growth factor receptor p75 expression was also significantly reduced in women with hormonally treated endometriosis compared with women with untreated endometriosis. Thus, hormonal treatment can significantly reduce nerve fiber density in endometrium and myometrium in women with endometriosis (Tokushige *et al* 2007).

Endometriosis is associated with low follicular-fluid BDNF levels, and diminished ovarian reserve is associated with increased follicular-fluid NGF levels. Follicular-fluid neurotrophin levels were determined in women undergoing assisted reproductive techniques for different etiologies of infertility in a prospective observational study. Women with a history of endometriosis have significantly lower follicular-fluid BDNF levels compared with women with male-factor (control) infertility. Women with diminished ovarian reserve have significantly higher levels of nerve growth factor (NGF) compared with women with male-factor infertility. Follicular-fluid BDNF levels tend to be lower in patients with endometriosis and diminished ovarian reserve and to be higher in patients with polycystic ovarian syndrome. Interestingly, NGF concentrations follow the opposite trend. But, follicular-fluid NT-3 concentrations are similar in women with different etiologies of infertility (Buyuk *et al* 2008).

Polycystic Ovaries

Even though it is impossible to reproduce human PCOS in an animal model, murine models may provide important leads. Studies on adult normal cycling rats found that a single intramuscular (i.m.) injection of estradiol valerate (EV) causes acyclicity and formation of PCO. The EV-induced rat PCO model reflects some endocrinological and morphological characteristics of human PCOS, and it is assumed that activity in the ovarian sympathetic nerves is higher than in normal rats. This is evidenced by an early increase in ovarian levels of norepinephrine (NE), an enhanced release of NE from ovarian nerve terminals, an increased activity of the catecholamine synthesis-limiting enzyme tyrosine hydroxylase (TH), and down-regulation of β2-adrenoceptors (ARs) in theca-interstitial cells (Manni *et al* 2006). Anti-NGF treatment in the PCO group restored all changes in mRNA and protein content, except that of alpha1b-AR and TrkA mRNAs, to control levels.

An increase in sympathetic outflow to the ovary proceeds, by several weeks, the appearance of cysts, suggesting the involvement of a neurogenic component in the pathology of this ovarian dysfunction. This change in sympathetic tone is related to an augmented production of ovarian NGF, and this abnormally elevated production of NGF contributes to the formation of ovarian cysts induced by EV (Lara *et al* 2000). Intraovarian administration of a neutralizing antiserum to NGF in conjunction with an antisense oligodeoxynucleotide to p75 NGFR, via Alzet osmotic minipumps, restored estrous cyclicity and ovulatory capacity in a majority of EV-treated rats. These functional changes were accompanied by restoration of the number of antral follicles per ovary that had been depleted by EV and a significant reduction in the number of both precystic follicles and follicular cysts. The hyperactivation of ovarian sympathetic nerves seen in EV-induced PCO is related to an overproduction of NGF and its low affinity receptor in the gland. Activation of this neurotrophic-neurogenic regulatory loop is a component of the pathological process by which EV induces cyst formation and anovulation in rodents. A similar alteration in neurotrophic input to the ovary might contribute to the etiology and/or maintenance of the PCO syndrome in humans.

Electro-acupuncture (EA) is known to reduce hyperactivity in the sympathetic nervous system. Repeated EA treatments in PCO rats resulted in concentrations of NGF in the ovaries that were significantly lower than those in non-EA-treated PCO rats but were within a normal range that did not differ from those in the untreated groups. The results provided support for the theory that EA inhibits hyperactivity in the sympathetic nervous system (Stener-Victorin *et al* 2000).

Possible role of EA in the regulation of ovarian responsiveness to sympathetic inputs depicts a possible complementary therapeutic approach to overcoming sympathetic-related anovulation in women with PCOS (Manni *et al* 2005, Bai *et al* 2004).

5 weeks of voluntary exercise influence ovarian morphology and the expression of sympathetic markers in the EV-induced PCO rat model. The results obtained indicated that ovarian morphology was almost normalised in the PCO exercise group; NGF mRNA and protein concentrations were normalised in the PCO exercise group; high numbers of NGF receptor expressing cells in PCO ovaries were lowered by exercise. Beneficial effect of regular exercise, as a modulator of ovarian sympathetic innervation was observed in the prevention and treatment of human PCOS (Manni *et al* 2005).

Breast Cancer

NGF is able to stimulate the proliferation of breast cancer cells (MCF-7 and MDA-MB-231 cell lines). But, it is unable to stimulate growth of normal breast epithelial cells (NBEC) (Descamps *et al* 1998). In cells expressing low levels of TrkA such as breast carcinoma cells, NGF must recruit other overexpressed receptors such as p185 (HER2) in order to generate a biological signal that can induce breast cancer cell growth (Tagliabue *et al* 2000). The antiestrogen drug tamoxifen (TAM) inhibited NGF-induced MCF-7 cell proliferation and trkA (NGFR) phosphorylation in a concentration-related fashion. The effect of TAM seemed to be estrogen receptor-independent (Chiarenza *et al* 2000). Two distinct signaling pathways are required for NGF activity and confirm the roles played by p75NTR and NF-kappaB in the activation of the survival pathway in breast cancer cells (Descamps *et al* 2001). NGF receptors and signaling are thus looking increasingly promising as potential drug targets for breast cancer. Physiological relevance of NGF in breast cancer and its potential interest as a marker and therapeutic target is fast gaining ground (Dollé *et al* 2003).

Serous Ovarian Carcinoma

Correlation between expression and activation of the high-affinity nerve growth factor (NGF) receptor TrkA, cell cycle protein expression, and disease outcome in serous ovarian carcinoma was analyzed by Davidson *et al* (2003) in malignant effusions and corresponding solid tumors in serous ovarian carcinoma.

In the ovary, NT including NGF can help in follicular maturation and ovulation by inducing the FSH receptor (FSHR). Current literature shows that perimenopausal ovarian surface epithelium (OSE) can also express FSHR. By G protein link, this FSHR is capable of precipitating neoplasia of OSE, which is the commonest in the ovary. NTs may be implicated as the cause of this aberrant expression of FSHR in OSE. By central action NT can lower serum FSH, as is found in postmenopausal ovarian cancer. Thus, NGF deregulates expression of FSHR in OSE and secretion of FSH from the pituitary. This phenomenon may hold the key to the hitherto unexplained carcinogenic process of sporadic epithelial ovarian cancer (Bose 2005).

NGF and trkA proteins were absent or found in very low levels in normal ovarian surface epithelium (OSE), whereas they were highly expressed in epithelial cells of EOC. Additionally, NGF stimulated the expression of VEGF isoforms in cancer explants. The effect was dose-dependent and inhibited by a NGF antibody and by K252a, a trk receptor inhibitor. This strongly suggests an autocrine role of NGF in EOC (Campos *et al* 2007). Thus, blocking neurotrophin action could be a therapeutic target in treating ovarian cancer.

Epidermal growth factor receptor, EGFR and TrkB crosstalk each other in response to EGF and BDNF, leading to cell survival pathway activation in ovarian cancer cells. A combination of inhibitors of both receptors with cell survival pathway inhibitors may provide a better outcome in the clinical treatment of ovarian cancer (Qiu *et al* 2006). NGF receptors probably signal via MAPK-independent pathways in ovarian carcinoma (Ødegaard *et al* 2007). Follitropin receptor knockout (FORKO) mice are sterile and have age-dependent abnormalities including increased ovarian tumor incidence. To explore why atrophic ovaries of FORKO mice become tumorigenic later in life, gene expression profile was done by microarray at different ages showing unexpected ovarian expression of glial cell line-derived neurotrophic factor, GDNF and its bimodal regulation (Aravindakshan *et al* 2006). Though evidence for GDNF up-regulation in GC tumors and a potential role for androgen were suggested, typical epithelial ovarian cancer might have different pathology.

Conclusion

Using sophisticated in vivo and in vitro techniques it is becoming possible to search for many NGF target cells including those of reproductive system. With multimodal approach NGF target cells are located in the immune system, neuroendocrine and hematopoietic cell lines thus revealing other as yet uncovered roles of this growth factor. Pharmacological agents that modify NGF gene expression or processing acting on the same path as those involved in the regulation of the synthesis and release of NGF could come out in near future by which it will be possible to interfere many endocrinal, immunological and other biological processes to our advantage.

Acknowledgements: nil
Disclosure of interests: nil
Contribution to authorship: single authorship
Details of ethics approval: not applicable
Funding: self funded review study

References

Akasu, F; Tagawa, Y; Shimada, H. Promoting effects of the combined administration of nerve growth promoting factor (NGF) and human chorionic gonadotropin (HCG) on the ovaries and uteri of immature mice. *Acta Obstet Gynaeco.l Jpn.* 1970 Jul; 17(3), 179-85

Anaf, V; Simon, P; El Nakadi, I; Fayt, I; et al. Hyperalgesia, nerve infiltration and nerve growth factor expression in deep adenomyotic nodules, peritoneal and ovarian endometriosis. *Hum. Reprod.* 2002 Jul; 17(7),1895-900.

Anesetti, G; Lombide, P; D'Albora, H; Ojeda SR. Intrinsic neurons in the human ovary. *Cell Tissue Res.* 2001 Nov; 306(2), 231-7.

Aravindakshan, J; Chen, XL; Sairam, MR. Age-dependent bimodal GDNF regulation during ovarian tumorigenesis in follitropin receptor mutant mice.: *Biochem. Biophys. Res. Commun.* 2006 Dec 15; 351(2), 507-13.

Ayer-LeLievre C, Olson L, Ebendal T, Hallböök F, Persson H.. Nerve growth factor mRNA and protein in the testis and epididymis of mouse and rat. *Proc. Natl. Acad. Sci. USA.* 1988 Apr;85(8):2628-32.

Bai, YH; Lim, SC; Song, CH; Bae, CS; et al. Electro-acupuncture reverses nerve growth factor abundance in experimental polycystic ovaries in the rat. *Gynecol. Obstet. Invest.* 2004; 57(2), 80-5.

Beer, DJ; Matloff, SM; Rocklin, RE. The influence of histamine on immune and inflammatory responses. *Adv. Immunol.* 1984; 35, 209-215.

Bianchi, R; Brozzi, F; and Donato, R. Increases Proliferation in PC12 Neuronal Cells and Reduces Their Responsiveness to Nerve Growth Factor via Akt Activation. *J. Biol. Chem.* 2005, 280 (6), Feb 11, 4402–4414,

Bigon, E; Soranzo, C; Minozzi, C; Skaper, SD; Callegaro, L. Large scale purification and immunological characterization of human placental nerve growth factor. *Neurochem. Res.* 1990 Dec, 15(12), 1197-202.

Bose, CK. Nerve growth factor, follicle stimulating hormone receptor and epithelial ovarian cancer. *Med. Hypotheses.* 2004, 63(5), 917-8.

Bose, CK. Role of nerve growth factor and FSH receptor in epithelial ovarian cancer. *Reprod. Biomed. Online.* 2005 Aug, 11(2), 194-7.

Brauer, MM; Shockley, KP; Chávez, R; Richeri, A; et al. The role of NGF in pregnancy-induced degeneration and regeneration of sympathetic nerves in the guinea pig uterus. *J. Auton. Nerv. Syst.* 2000 Feb 14, 79(1), 19-27

Bryman, I; Norström, A; Dahlström, A; Lindblom, B. Immunohistochemical evidence for preserved innervation of the human cervix during pregnancy. *Gynecol. Obstet Invest.* 1987, 24(2), 73-9.

Buyuk, E; Seifer, DB. Follicular-fluid neurotrophin levels in women undergoing assisted reproductive technology for different etiologies of infertility. *Fertil Steril.* 2008 Jan 25 [Epub ahead of print]

Campos, X; Muñoz, Y; Selman, A; Yazigi, R; et al. Nerve growth factor and its high-affinity receptor trkA participate in the control of vascular endothelial growth factor expression in epithelial ovarian cancer. *Gynecol. Oncol.* 2007 Jan, 104(1), 168-75.

Chao, MV; Bothwell, M. Neurotrophins: to cleave or not to cleave. *Neuron* 2002, 33, 9–12

Chapman, CA; Banks, BE; Carstairs, JR; Pearce, FL; Vernon, CA. The preparation of nerve growth factor from the prostate of the guinea-pig and isolation of immunogenically pure material from the mouse submandibular gland. *FEBS Lett.* 1979 Sep 15, 105(2), 341-4.

Chiarenza, A; Lazarovici, P; Lempereur, L; Cantarella, G; et al.Tamoxifen inhibits nerve growth factor-induced proliferation of the human breast cancerous cell line MCF-7. *Cancer Res.* 2001 Apr 1, 61(7), 3002-8.

Chiarenza, A; Lazarovici, P; Lempereur, L; Cantarella, G; et al. Tamoxifen inhibits nerve growth factor-induced proliferation of the human breast cancerous cell line MCF-7. *Cancer Res.* 2001 Apr 1, 61(7), 3002-8.

Davidson, B; Reich, R; Lazarovici, P; Nesland, JM; et al. Expression and activation of the nerve growth factor receptor TrkA in serous ovarian carcinoma. *Clin. Cancer Res.* 2003 Jun, 9(6), 2248-59.

Descamps, S; Lebourhis, X; Delehedde, M; Boilly, B; Hondermarck, H. Nerve growth factor is mitogenic for cancerous but not normal human breast epithelial cells. *J. Biol. Chem.* 1998 Jul 3, 273(27), 16659-62.

Descamps, S; Toillon, RA; Adriaenssens, E; Pawlowski, V; et al. Nerve growth factor stimulates proliferation and survival of human breast cancer cells through two distinct signaling pathways. *J. Biol. Chem.* 2001 May 25, 276(21), 17864-70.

Dissen, GA; Hill, DF; Costa, ME; Les Dees, CW; Lara HE, Ojeda SR.A role for trkA nerve growth factor receptors in mammalian ovulation. *Endocrinology.* 1996 Jan, 137(1), 198-209.

Dissen, GA; Hill, DF; Costa, ME; Ma, YJ; Ojeda, SR. Nerve growth factor receptors in the peripubertal rat ovary. *Mol. Endocrinol.* 1991 Nov, 5(11), 1642-50.

Dissen, GA; Hirshfield, AN; Malamed, S; Ojeda, SR. Expression of neurotrophins and their receptors in the mammalian ovary is developmentally regulated: changes at the time of folliculogenesis. *Endocrinology.* 1995 Oct, 136(10), 4681-92.

Dollé, L; El Yazidi-Belkoura, I; Adriaenssens, E; Nurcombe, V; Hondermarck, H; Nerve growth factor overexpression and autocrine loop in breast cancer cells. *Oncogene.* 2003 Aug 28, 22(36), 5592-601.

Emanuele, E; Politi, P; Bianchi, M; Minoretti, P; et al. Raised plasma nerve growth factor levels associated with early-stage romantic love. *Psychoneuroendocrinology.* 2006 Apr, 31(3), 288-94.

Gazzolo, D; Marinoni E, Di Iorio, R; Lituania, M; et al. High maternal blood S100B concentrations in pregnancies complicated by intrauterine growth restriction and intraventricular hemorrhage. *Clin. Chem.* 2006 May;52(5):819-26.

Goldstein, LD; Reynolds, CP; Perez-Polo, JR. Isolation of human nerve growth factor from placental tissue. *Neurochem. Res.* 1978 Apr, 3(2), 175-83.

Green, AR; Edwards, RE; Greaves, P; White, IN. Comparison of the effect of oestradiol, tamoxifen and raloxifene on nerve growth factor-alpha expression in specific neonatal mouse uterine cell types using laser capture microdissection. *J. Mol. Endocrinol.* 2003 Feb, 30(1), 1-11.

Green, AR; Styles, JA; Parrott, EL; Gray, D; et al. Neonatal tamoxifen treatment of mice leads to adenomyosis but not uterine cancer. *Exp. Toxicol. Pathol.* 2005 Mar; 56(4-5): 255-63

Harper, GP; Barde, YA; Burnstock, G; Carstairs, JR; et al. Guinea pig prostate is a rich source of nerve growth factor. *Nature* 279, 160 - 162 (10 May 1979).

Krizsan-Agbas, D; Pedchenko, T; Hasan, W; Smith, PG. Oestrogen regulates sympathetic neurite outgrowth by modulating brain derived neurotrophic factor synthesis and release by the rodent uterus. *Eur. J. Neurosci.* 2003 Nov, 18(10), 2760-65.

Lara, HE; Dissen, GA; Leyton, V; Paredes, A; et al. An increased intraovarian synthesis of nerve growth factor and its low affinity receptor is a principal component of steroid-induced polycystic ovary in the rat. *Endocrinology.* 2000 Mar, 141(3), 1059-72.

Lara, HE; McDonald, JK; Ojeda, SR. Involvement of nerve growth factor in female sexual development. *Endocrinology.* 1990 Jan, 126(1), 364-75.

Levi-Montalcini, R; Hamburger, V. Selective growth stimulating effects of mouse sarcoma on the sensory and sympathetic nervous system of the chick embryo. *J. Exp. Zool.* 1951 Mar, 116(2), 321-61.

Levi-Montalcini R. The Nerve Growth Factor. *Ann. N Y Acad. Sci.* 1964 Oct 9, 118, 149-70.

Lobos, E; Gebhardt, C; Kluge, A; and Spanel-Borowski, K. Expression of Nerve Growth Factor (NGF) Isoforms in the Rat Uterus during Pregnancy: Accumulation of Precursor proNGF. *Endocrinology.* 2005, 146 (4), 1922-1929

Lommatzsch, M; Hornych, K; Zingler, C; Schuff-Werner, P; et al. Maternal serum concentrations of BDNF and depression in the perinatal period. *Psychoneuroen docrinology.* 2006 Apr, 31(3), 388-94.

Luppi, P; Levi-Montalcini, R; Bracci-Laudiero, L; Bertolini, A; et al. NGF is released into plasma during human pregnancy: an oxytocin-mediated response? *Neuroreport.* 1993 Aug, 4(8), 1063-5.

Malamitsi-Puchner, A; Nikolaou, KE; Economou, E; Boutsikou, M; et al. Intrauterine growth restriction and circulating neurotrophin levels at term. *Early Hum. Dev.* 2007 Jul, 83(7), 465-9.

Manni, L; Cajander, S; Lundeberg, T; Naylor, AS; et al. Effect of exercise on ovarian morphology and expression of nerve growth factor and alpha(1)- and beta(2)-adrenergic receptors in rats with steroid-induced polycystic ovaries. *J. Neuroendocrinol.* 2005 Dec;17(12):846-58.

Manni, L; Holmäng, A; Cajander, S; Lundeberg, T; et al. Effect of anti-NGF on ovarian expression of alpha1- and beta2-adrenoceptors, TrkA, p75NTR, and tyrosine hydroxylase in rats with steroid-induced polycystic ovaries. *Am. J. Physiol. Regul. Integr. Comp Physiol.* 2006 Mar, 290(3), 826-35.

Manni, L; Lundeberg, T; Holmäng, A; Aloe, L; Stener-Victorin, E. Effect of electro-acupuncture on ovarian expression of alpha (1)- and beta (2)-adrenoceptors, and p75 neurotrophin receptors in rats with steroid-induced polycystic ovaries. *Reprod. Biol. Endocrinol.* 2005 Jun 7, 3, 21

Martocchia, A; Sigala, S; Proietti, A; D'Urso, R; et al. Sex-related variations in serum nerve growth factor concentration in humans. *Neuropeptides.* 2002 Dec, 36(6), 391-5.

Mayerhofer, A; Dissen, GA; Parrott, JA; Hill, DF; et al. Involvement of nerve growth factor in the ovulatory cascade: trkA receptor activation inhibits gap junctional communication between thecal cells. *Endocrinology.* 1996 Dec, 137(12), 5662-70.

Mechsner, S; Schwarz, J; Thode, J; Loddenkemper, C; et al. Growth-associated protein 43-positive sensory nerve fibers accompanied by immature vessels are located in or near peritoneal endometriotic lesions. *Fertil Steril.* 2007 Sep, 88(3), 581-7.

Naves, FJ; Vázquez, MT; José, IS; Martínez-Almagro, A; Vega, JA. Pregnancy-induced denervation of the human uterine artery correlates with local decrease of NGF and TrkA. *Ital. J. Anat. Embryol. 1998*,103(4 Suppl 1), 279-90.

Ødegaard, E; Staff, AC; Abeler, VM; Kopolovic, J; et al. The activated nerve growth factor receptor p-TrkA is selectively expressed in advanced-stage ovarian carcinoma. *Hum. Pathol.* 2007 Jan, 38(1), 140-6.

Ojeda, SR; Dissen, GA; Junier, MP. Neurotrophic factors and female sexual development. *Front Neuroendocrinol.* 1992 Apr, 13(2), 120-62.

Ojeda, SR; Romero, C; Tapia, V; Dissen, GA. Neurotrophic and cell-cell dependent control of early follicular development. *Mol. Cell Endocrinol.* 2000 May 25, 163(1-2), 67-71.

Qiu, L; Zhou, C; Sun, Y; Di, W; et al. Crosstalk between EGFR and TrkB enhances ovarian cancer cell migration and proliferation. *Int. J. Oncol.* 2006 Oct, 29(4), 1003-11

Ren, L; Medan, MS; Weng, Q; Jin, W; et al. J Immunolocalization of nerve growth factor (NGF) and its receptors (TrkA and p75LNGFR) in the reproductive organs of Shiba goats. *Reprod. Dev.* 2005 Jun, 51(3), 399-404.

Richard, A; McColl, SR; Pelletier, G. Interleukin-4 and nerve growth factor can act as cofactors for interleukin-3-induced histamine production in human umbilical cord blood cells in serum-free culture. *Br. J. Haematol.* 1992 May, 81(1), 6-11.

Romero, C; Paredes, A; Dissen, GA; Ojeda, SR. Nerve growth factor induces the expression of functional FSH receptors in newly formed follicles of the rat ovary. *Endocrinology.* 2002 Apr, 143(4), 1485-94.

Stener-Victorin, E; Lundeberg, T; Cajander, S; Aloe, L; et al. Steroid-induced polycystic ovaries in rats: effect of electro-acupuncture on concentrations of endothelin-1 and nerve growth factor (NGF), and expression of NGF mRNA in the ovaries, the adrenal glands, and the central nervous system. *Reprod. Biol. Endocrinol.* 2003 Apr 8, 1, 33.

Tagliabue, E; Castiglioni, F; Ghirelli, C; Modugno, M; et al. Nerve growth factor cooperates with p185(HER2) in activating growth of human breast carcinoma cells. *J. Biol. Chem.* 2000 Feb 25, 275(8), 5388-94.

Tokushige, N; Markham, R; Russell, P; Fraser, IS. Nerve fibres in peritoneal endometriosis. *Hum. Reprod.* 2006 Nov, 21(11), 3001-7.

Tokushige, N; Markham, R; Russell, P; Fraser, IS. Effects of hormonal treatment on nerve fibers in endometrium and myometrium in women with endometriosis. *Fertil Steril.* 2007 Nov 30 [Epub ahead of print].

Tometten, M; Blois, S; Arck, PC. Nerve growth factor in reproductive biology: link between the immune, endocrine and nervous system? *Chem. Immunol. Allergy*. 2005, 89, 135-48.

Tometten, M; Blois, S; Kuhlmei, A; Stretz, A; Klapp, BF; Arck, PC. Nerve growth factor translates stress response and subsequent murine abortion via adhesion molecule-dependent pathways. *Biol. Reprod.* 2006 Apr, 74(4), 674-83.

Tometten, M; Klapp, BF; Joachim, R; Fest, S; et al. Nerve growth factor and its functional receptor TrkA are up-regulated in murine decidual tissue of stress-triggered and substance P-mediated abortion. *Am. J. Reprod. Immunol.* 2004 Jan;51(1):86-93.

Toti, P; Ciarmela, P; Florio, P; Volpi, N; et al. Human placenta and fetal membranes express nerve growth factor mRNA and protein. *J. Endocrinol. Invest.* 2006 Apr, 29(4), 337-41.

Tskitishvili, E; Komoto, Y; Temma-Asano, K; Hayashi, S; Kinugasa, Y; et al. S100B protein expression in the amnion and amniotic fluid in pregnancies complicated by pre-eclampsia. *Mol. Hum. Reprod.* 2006 Dec;12(12):755-61.

Varol, FG; Duchemin, AM; Neff, NH; Hadjiconstantinou, M. Nerve growth factor (NGF) and NGF mRNA change in rat uterus during pregnancy. *Neurosci. Lett.* 2000 Nov 10, 294(1), 58-62.

Index

A

F

G

H

I

N

Q

R

S

T

U

V

W

X

Y